GAME ON

GAME ON
A Team Approach to Cancer

MISTI AND JAY COKER

Pep Rally Press
www.personalpeprally.org
misticoker@gmail.com

ISBN: 978-0-9972312-9-8

Front cover photograph: The true definition of a team is
the photo on the front cover. Stringer's senior players
have been with him since day one of his cancer diagnosis.
These young men have cared for him on and off the
court. They are the reason many days that he would get
up and go. Stringer has taught them much more than just
basketball; he has taught them many life lessons. One of
the most significant lessons is this: "Don't give up!" This
picture was taken after these seniors finished the ENDURE
THE DIRT 5K Adventure Mud Run located on the farm
ground around Mack's Prairie Wings in Stuttgart,
Arkansas. The family of Stringer's wife, Lauren, created
this race, and all proceeds go to encourage, motivate, and
educate cancer patients and their families. You can learn
more at **www.personalpeprally.org.**

Book design: H. K. Stewart
Illustration on page 40: Nancy Duke

All Biblical quotations are from the New International
Version unless otherwise noted.

Printed in the United States of America.
This book is printed on archival-quality paper that meets
requirements of the American National Standard for
Information Sciences, Permanence of Paper, Printed
Library Materials, ANSI Z39.48-1984.

To our son-in-law **Marc Stringer**
and our daughter **Lauren Coker Stringer**

Your strength amazes us every day. Through the fight, you have kept your faith, even when it wasn't easy. You have pressed on through the pregame, the game, and now the postgame. Your journey is going to encourage and motivate many people who have been given a cancer diagnosis.

We love you,
Mom and Dad

DISCLAIMER

This book contains information that is intended to help the reader be better informed when diagnosed with cancer. It is not designed to be a substitute for medical advice from a licensed physician. Always consult with your doctor to determine your individual needs. This information is not to be construed as legal advice. Always seek appropriate counsel when dealing with personal situations.

We have made every effort to ensure that the information in this book was correct at press time.

Contents

Author's Note

After I completed all of the necessary research and interviews with cancer patients, cancer families, and their friends, I wanted to find an influential football coach who had experienced cancer to write the Foreword. I searched out several who led me NO WHERE! I started to doubt whether I was even to finish this endeavor. I questioned God and thought maybe I should move on to something else. That is when God stepped in.

Jay encouraged me to go to the Rotary sports luncheon. I didn't want to go at all, but I went. Jay told me that Fitz Hill would be speaking, and he thought I would enjoy his talk. At the time I had no idea who Fitz Hill was, and my brain was saying, "I have too much to do to go sit through a boring lunch."

I sat through lunch, and then it was time for this Fitz Hill guy to begin his motivational spiel on what would bring me to tears and change my mindset. Fitz started speaking and said that this talk was for the young people in the room, the ones who think they can't move forward. Within the first three minutes of his speech, I knew Fitz was the guy. He spoke about his father being diagnosed with cancer and how it changed him. Yep, God had spoken to me through Fitz.

When the luncheon was over, I wrote a note on a little piece of paper that had my name and number. I approached Fitz crying—yes crying, and those who know me know I'm not the crying type. I told him I was working on a project and I thought he could help me. If he was interested in learning more, give me a call.

The rest is history, and Fitz and I have been working together for over a year. Fitz is one of the most God-led people I know. Every time I visit with him, he lifts my spirits and reminds me that God is in control and it is all in His timing. Fitz has taught me that by walking with God and by having a WANT TO attitude, much can be accomplished.

God showed out that day over a year ago at a Rotary lunch leading me to Fitz.

Misti Coker

Fitz Hill *is a former American football player and coach and college administrator. He has played a role in every part of football from the high school level to the college level. Fitz also was in the military serving during the Gulf War and participating in Desert Shield and Desert Storm. He was promoted to first lieutenant and received the Bronze Star and Commendation Medal. Above all else, Fitz is a devout Christian putting God first in everything he does.*

Foreword

Dr. Fitz Hill

It was early spring 1980 at Arkadelphia High School in southwest Arkansas when a student worker walked into my classroom and told the teacher that I was needed in the principal's office. My mother was the school's registrar so I thought to myself, what have I done for my mother to send someone from the office to get me? What I didn't realize was that my life would never be the same again upon seeing my mother. My life as I knew it for the past 15 years was about to change…forever.

As I proceeded into the principal's office, I immediately noticed a grave look of concern on my mother's face and instantly thought to myself, I'm in big trouble. My mother took me in the assistant principal's office and closed the door and told me to sit down. She needed to tell me something. My heart was pounding, and I started thinking about everything I could have possibly done wrong over the last week. My mother, Mary S. Hill, told me that my daddy, her husband, James Omon Hill, needed to be taken immediately to see a doctor in Little Rock because, "Your Daddy has been diagnosed with cancer."

Cancer…a word that I had heard before, but it really was a foreign language to me. However, my mother was not a medical language translator, so I sat there confused, baffled at the grave expression on her face, and wondered what this meant for our family and me. I did not really understand the impact of the disease because I had never had a close family member or even known anyone personally who had cancer or had died from the disease. I just remember feeling as if I were dreaming as my Mother was trying to explain to me that Daddy was really sick and we had to leave the school immediately and take him to Little Rock because local doctors couldn't treat him. She checked me out of school, and we departed expeditiously.

We would discover that Daddy had been sick with cancer for a while, but it was difficult to diagnose because he was having his teeth extracted, which impacted his appetite and changed his normal eating habits. We had assumed he was losing weight because his gums were healing from the teeth extractions and he was unable to eat solid food because he had yet to receive his dentures, and that was why he had lost a lot of weight. We would soon find out that having his teeth removed did contribute to his weight loss, but that was *not* the real problem. Daddy was suffering from some serious issues associated with cancer and his illness was exacerbated due to the fact that he had not been going to the doctor to get regular check-ups to catch the disease in its early stages.

The emotional and physical toll that cancer can have on families is rarely understood until a loved one is diagnosed and you observe first hand their health deteriorating little by little each day in front of your eyes. I prayed every moment for a miracle cure for my daddy and hoped on each doctor's visit that we would receive encouraging news. But you never know how the cancer is going to respond to the medical treatment, so you just keep praying to God for a miracle, and you get mad when you don't think God is listening and you feel as if he refuses to answer your prayers and heal your loved ones.

That's what I felt with my father. Even today, when I hear certain music that takes me back to the early 80s, I can frequently associate those memories with my dad's cancer. Those images are still fresh and real in my mind. and to be quite honest, so is the pain. But somehow you learn to cope with the pain, but without God, I'm not sure you ever truly heal.

During my first 15 years of life, my daddy was the epitome of being physically fit. I joined him on Saturday mornings cutting grass at the young age of seven years old while also helping him clean the medical office of one of the doctors in the community. At the age of 12, I started working with him at the bottling plant where I developed my work ethic by hanging out and imitating him making Mr. Cola, Sun Drop, and NuGrape sodas. However, the day Daddy was diagnosed with cancer, he never worked another day at the bottling plant or pushed another lawn mower to cut grass.

Yep, all of that changed after my daddy had surgery to remove the cancer from his stomach, which required the removal of most of his stomach. I watched Daddy battle cancer and return to his original weight. He was even able to be employed again for the purpose of trying to support his family. Things had really gotten tight financially due to the fact that we went from a two household income to one and the disability benefits were limited. Consequently, Daddy wanted to work to support his family, and he decided that he could work as a janitor making minimum wage so he could bring home some needed funds to help support his family. This is how cancer changes things for families, and this is what I mean when I said that life as you knew is never the same when a doctor tells the family that their loved has cancer.

Christmas of 1982 remains a fresh tattoo in my memory. It was the last Christmas we would celebrate with Daddy. The cancer returned requiring a second surgery resulting in a colostomy and this time chemotherapy to battle the cancerous cells. Daddy was defeated in his battle with the disease and perished from this earth a couple days after Thanksgiving in November of 1983 at the age of 52.

You don't realize how much you cherish being with someone you love until they are not here to celebrate the holidays and special occasions with you anymore. Cancer does not discriminate, and in my case the deadly disease has been a dominating force in wrecking my family. Eleven years later my brother was diagnosed with cancer and only lived a very short time with the disease resulting in him departing this earth at the tender age of 40. The impact of his death sent shock waves through his family, and in my personal opinion, his family was negatively impacted in ways similar to how the death of my father emotionally traumatized his wife and three sons.

Why is this relevant? When cancer strikes and blindsides your family, you need a *team* of first responders who can help you navigate the negatives associated with the disease. I can tell you first hand, the death of our father devastated the three boys that James Omon Hill had raised and supported. Not to mention the fact that six weeks after we buried my father, my mother had an aneurysm in church resulting in her becoming a hemiplegic without the ability to walk or talk for the rest of her life. It is believed that the three years of emotional stress my mother experienced while taking care of my daddy's daily needs associated with cancer took a mental and physical toll on her. Often times when you are dealing with family members with terminal cancer, you neglect the treatment you need for yourself. This is what we assumed happened with my mother, and this also impacted my brothers and me. Cancer burdened our entire family, and the ripple effect was devastating to our family, and according to my current family, they are still feeling the shrapnel of the emotional trauma I experienced dealing with the fallout of family illnesses associated with this fatal disease.

If my life were being described in terms of a football game, I would say that cancer intercepted my life by blitzing and blindsiding my daddy and brother by taking their lives. This set back caused me to fumble spiritually in many ways and lose sight of the life God purposed for me. However, I do believe that God will send teammates to help you take the setbacks of life associated with the illness of cancer to create a game plan for a comeback. But trusting in the Lord is how you make significant plays of emotional restoration… not leaning on your own understanding and finding temporary ways to cope with your pain when going through family crisis associated with cancer. God is a healer and comforter. Trust Him. Trust Him.

INTRODUCTION

We want to begin by saying, "We are sorry." Our family truly empathizes with the emotions you are having. On July 1, 2016, our daughter Lauren and her husband, Marc ("Stringer"), heard the words, "YOU HAVE CANCER" when he was diagnosed with esophageal cancer. Just like you and your loved ones, we have been inflicted with this disease. During the weeks following the cancer diagnosis, we sat many days in waiting rooms. It was at this time that we realized how many people are affected by cancer. Our minds raced from one emotion to another.

We, like you, have been thrown into a storm. We have been pushing forward through the wind, the rain, and even on some days more hazardous weather. There are the questions: Why did this happen? What could have prevented this? What is next? Some days the storms seemed too much to bear, so forceful we couldn't see.

Some of the questions we had answers for, some questions would never be answered, but then there were the questions we knew someone could answer. The problem was that you don't call your oncologist in the middle of the night. So where did we turn? We turned to others who had cancer or were cancer survivors.

17

We began to devise a plan to gather as much information as we could from cancer patients, their families, and their friends.

People who have withstood the storms are the best to help those in the storm.

We began to understand that there is a purpose for all situations and God was going to use this circumstance for good.

At the beginning of our journey, Lauren asked her dad, Jay, if he would send Marc a motivating text. Since Marc is a coach, Jay used sports analogies and ended with the words GAME ON! These two words sparked the inspiration for this book.

Our main purpose for the book *Game On!* is to help people who have been given a cancer diagnosis. We want to share the information we have gathered from our experiences and from other cancer patients' experiences about the ins and outs of a cancer journey.

Our prayer is that you find peace, comfort, and answers located within the pages of *Game On!*

From this point on, YOU ARE THE WINNER; you are going to rise to the occasion. Cancer isn't going to define you; you are going to define cancer. GAME ON!

Misti Coker

CONFIDENT CHALLENGE

Just like in athletics, you have to have confidence in your team. Your doctors, nurses, friends, and family—that's your team now. Follow their plan and embrace it. Positive thoughts produce positive outcomes. Cancer is your opponent. Never fear it. Fear is a lack of faith. Trust in your team, yourself, the Lord, and His plan. Your test results will be your scouting report. From this, you'll overcome your opponent. Maintain confidence and a positive, prayerful attitude. Those around you will feed off you. You will gain more power as these positive thoughts multiply among your team. Hold your head high and meet your opponent and challenge head on.

Believe in yourself, because we all do. We will beat this.

GAME ON!

Jay Coker

CANCER IS YOUR OPPONENT. NEVER FEAR IT. FEAR IS A LACK OF FAITH.

19

1.
Headed In

If you are from Arkansas and know anything about high school football, you have heard the name George Burke. He was a one-of-a-kind high school coach who captured so many wins, he made high school history. Burke was a great coach because he related all football lessons to life lessons. My husband was on Burke's state championship Ricebird team in 1982. Through the years, my daughters and I have heard quotes and phrases that Coach Burke imprinted on the brains of his players.

Dodd McCollum, who was on the state championship team with my husband, left Stuttgart and joined the Air Force. In his adult life, he, like many of his former fellow athletes, used quotes and lessons that he learned while playing football for Burke. Dodd said it best in an article written when Coach Burke passed away. Recalling the missions he flew overseas, Dodd wrote, "As my team was flying into battle, bombs were going off all around us. As I flew the plane, I quoted Coach Burke's words of wisdom: 'There is no turning back we are headed in!'"

TERRORIST

It is ironic that I began writing this book on September 11, 2016. Why, you may ask? Because cancer is like a terrorist.

Fifteen years before, terrorist hijackers had flown commercial planes into the World Trade Center in New York City and into the Pentagon in Washington, DC, and had crashed a fourth jet into the ground in Pennsylvania. When some of our family visited the 9-11 Memorial in New York, we learned many details of that horrific day in 2001.

The terrorists, who were members of al-Qaida, came to the United States and blended into society. They trained in several flight schools around the country. Even though the language was a barrier, they found a way to converse with others. They were in the flight school pictures, and they seemed to be part of the group. The instructors said there were no red flags.

Numerous pilots commented that they could not believe these amateur pilots could perform such advanced skills. The terrorists trained in small propeller planes, but then turned around and flew Boeings 757s without assistance. They were successful in navigating and hitting their target. How could these terrorists with mediocre skills fly these large aircraft and hit the bull's eye?

Cancer is much like a terrorist. Cancer cells blend in with normal cells. They are normal cells that turn into abnormal cells. These abnormal cells move in and try to fit in. Then they get to work. At first, they show no red flags, and they go undetected, but then it happens. Out of the blue, they attack. They attack the human body and cause devastation. They invade and spread, wreaking havoc throughout the body. Cancer hits the bull's eye.

Nine-11 affected many from different races, socio-economic groups, and generations; so does cancer. Cancer doesn't care about your age or your race. Cancer doesn't care if you live in New York or Arkansas. Cancer doesn't care if you have a family or if you are alone. Cancer doesn't care if you are rich or poor. Cancer doesn't care just as the terrorists didn't care. All they wanted to do was cause chaos and confusion.

Cancer, like a terrorist, has a job to do and it follows through. It drains us of peace and ignites fear. How many of you now look around as you board your airplane? Do you pray that TSA checks the person who may seem like a terrorist checking in ahead of you? Do you look at the Most Wanted Terrorist flyers and scope out every person in the airport? Call it paranoia, but that is what 9-11 did to us as Americans, and cancer does the same. We go into panic mode when we have a bump or a wound that won't heal. We read so much, hear so much, and know so much that we become paranoid we are next.

Nine-11 affected many people just like cancer affects many every day, every year. No one is immune to cancer. Terrorists can strike anywhere just as cancer can develop anywhere in the body. There are more than 100 different types of cancer. Cancer can be in the blood, in an organ, or even in tissue.

You are probably asking, "What causes this terrorist cell to be normal and then all of a sudden switch gears and become cancer?"

The Lord is my rock, my fortress and my deliverer; my God is my rock, in whom I take refuge, my shield and the horn of my salvation, my stronghold.

Psalm 18:2

23

CANCER, YOU
HAVE MESSED
WITH THE
WRONG TEAM!
WE ARE
HEADING IN,
AND WE ARE
NOT TURNING
BACK. WE ARE
READY TO MOVE
FULL SPEED
AHEAD—
GAME ON!

Some cancers are genetic, some are environmental, some are lifestyle factors, but for others, there is no reason for the cell to erupt into an overflowing volcano of hot lava invading your body.

Researchers don't have the answers to all the questions; however, we do know that cancer has a tremendous impact on our society—not only in the United States, but all over the world.

Now that we have discussed the cancer terrorist let's look at the basic facts about cancer.

- Cancer is an abnormal cell growing in your body that crowds out normal cells
- Cancer can be anywhere
- Cancer can be a tumor, lump, or a growth
- There are stages of cancer ranging from I-IV. The higher the stage, the more advanced the disease.
- Everyone is unique, so cancer treatments will be unique.
- Cancer is treated with chemotherapy, radiation, and surgery. You may have only one type of treatment; you may have a combination of two, or you may have all three. You may also be considered for a trial.
- You will probably never be able to answer the question, "Why me?"
- You are never alone in this game of cancer.

See the American Cancer Society's website at **www.cancer.org** for more information about cancer stages and treatments.

THOUGHTS

Stringer,
Esophageal Cancer Survivor

Don't give up.
Don't ever
give up

Jim Valvano

I always thought of myself as someone who could do anything by myself and usually wanted to. Going through cancer, however, has taught me that it is impossible to take on the task alone. Having a support group is key to surviving the fight. Everyone tells you how brave and how heroic you are during your battle, but I never felt that way. Others only saw the good. There were, and still are, countless times I didn't feel like getting up, wanted to give up, or just broke down and cried because of how tough a fight it is. Having a strong support system is key because it gives you someone to fight for you when you don't think you can. There will be days like that, trust me.

ASKING TO HELP

I'm not one to go and ask for help. Again, I have always been a person who wanted to do things on my own. So if someone you know is dealing with cancer, don't tell them, "Let me know if there is anything I can do." Instead, just do it—whether it's mowing their lawn, cleaning their house, taking out the trash, or bringing them a meal. It will be appreciated! When I was sick, I had someone mow my yard for me; people brought food. It helped take some of the burdens off my wife and just added to the feeling of support that we have behind us in our fight.

THE FIGHT

Cancer is the hardest thing I have ever been through. I played college football for five years, and I have always thought that going through Coach Mullins's preseason conditioning or practice sessions were some of the hardest things I have done—until cancer. Before my fight, I was doing a lot of reading and studying on mental toughness and mental psychology of sports. I don't know for sure, but I feel my athletic background helped me a great bit getting through the psychological aspects of the fight that cancer will throw at you. I was 33 at the time of my diagnosis and felt I was in the best shape of my life. When treatment hit me physically, it hit me like a hammer. It has taken a significant toll on my body from the year of treatment and surgery, even a year later I am still trying to get back a shred of what I had. It is happening, slowly.

Know that when you start your fight, the fight will last longer than the treatment. Cancer will attack you in every possible way, from physical to mental.

One thing that helped me get through cancer is that I met a lot of people, younger and older, while I was going through treatment, and many of them have fought cancer more than once or for a more extended period. Seeing and hearing their stories helped put this point into perspective for me. "Yes, I am going through a difficult fight, but I don't have it as bad as this person or that person. If they can do it for longer and harder, I can handle this."

26

ROUTINE

For me, sitting around ate at my mind. The worst thing I could do was sit around and think about cancer and the what if's. Staying in somewhat of my normal routine every day helped me deal with the negative thoughts of cancer—whether that was going to work or doing a little bit of my workouts. Anything that is in your normal day, DO IT.

Cancer tries to take things away from you. Not letting it take everything was key for me going through this. There will be days where you will want or need to just lie in bed, and that is fine to "recharge," but stay in your norm.

Cancer will change your thoughts, your fight, and your routine. You will have to change and adjust, but don't let cancer determine who you are. Cancer can't define you.

PERSONAL ESSAY

THE C WORD

Vickie—OBGYN, Daughter of Cancer Patient

The word was clear, but not the meaning. You know there's cancer, then there's CANCER. I've been a doctor for nearly 25 years, and I've been a chronically ill patient for three, so I've spent countless hours in doctor's offices and hospitals on both sides of the sheets. However, the overwhelming desire to run out the door was an unfamiliar feeling. Cancer, my dad has cancer.

No diagnosis is dreaded more. Though cancer isn't necessarily the worst disease, the word itself elicits gut-wrenching fear. It's a nasty word because cancer is an invasion. It occupies spaces it should not and not only invades organs, but families and souls as well.

Cancer is insidious. Lurking undetected in the body looking for an opportunity to push through boundaries and run rampant until it takes over. In its wake, it consumes strength, space, and nutrition.

Certain signs and warnings should not be ignored: lumps, sudden changes in energy or appetite or weight, and blood where it does not belong. Spiritual cancers are equally deadly, and similar warning signs should never go unchecked.

Lump

A lump is a mass or abnormal growth. Unclean thoughts, behaviors, and actions have no place in the life of a Christian either. Harboring unforgive-ness and jealousy occupies space in the heart where it does not belong. Sin invades the soul and destroys everything in its path.

Loss of Appetite

A healthy child of God hungers for the things of God. Sudden loss of appetite for prayer, Bible study, and fellowship with other believers is a red flag. When your spiritual appetite is gone, schedule an emergency appointment with the Great Physician.

Weight Loss

Lack of proper nutrition causes pounds to melt away. Cancer robs the body of essential nutrients and produces cachexia. There are plenty of things in this world that rob our souls of nutrition resulting in loss of fruit. If you have no joy, no love, no peace, check your heart.

PERSISTENT COUGH, BLEEDING, SORES

The mouth is a marker for the content of the heart. Bitter words flow from diseased hearts. A critical spirit and negative attitude are symptoms of a soul in need of a thorough exam.

FATIGUE

Cancer zaps strength and energy. Weariness in serving others indicates an imbalance of pouring out and pouring in. We need a continuous infusion from the life-giving source to prevent depletion.

GO TEAM

Early detection of cancer improves the likelihood of cure so never ignore warning signs—physical or spiritual. Still, cancer often sneaks in without visible signs, then it's a battle for life. My dad is ready to be done with chemotherapy, scans, procedures, and radiation, but this isn't a sprint. We can't focus on the finish line, but instead need to celebrate the mile markers. We are in for a long haul, and that is why we are huddling up and getting our game on!

PERSONAL ESSAY

THAT STEP

Alan—Colonel,
Author, Cancer Survivor

From 1983 until the present, I have taken many steps onto a battlefield. Being in the United States Army has led me into situations that were uncomfortable and at times felt uncontrollable. I stepped into these situations with my rifle and a palm pilot. I have been face to face with some of the most wanted villains from Saddam's regime and gone head to head to capture them. I have stepped in the line of duty making house calls to capture those that were out to destroy.

Though I have stepped onto the field numerous times, there was that one step that was different from any other.

As I was stepping onto a plane headed back to the Middle East I received a phone call from my doctor. He said, "Alan you can't get on that plane. You have cancer."

Many years I had been fighting for my country, but now I was fighting for me. I had never worried that I might lose my life while taking on a terrorist, but cancer was a different adversary. I had many hours and years of studying my opponent. I had learned strategies to capture them, to talk to them, to understand them. I knew to win I had to be respected and for that to happen, I had to learn about the culture and have cultural interactions. Winning the hearts and minds of the people in Iraq was crucial to our success.

In all my training, not one training event focused on the type of opponent I had to face now. There was no way to gain the respect of cancer. Cancer was a villain that I was not trained to go up against.

Even though my doctor urged me to stay in the U.S., I took that step and stepped on the plane headed overseas. I was going to fight this battle in the area where I had been fighting with terrorists for years.

Since I had learned the culture and gained respect from many, I had people who were ready to help me fight my opponent. They had studied their opponent and knew the best strategies to help destroy the cancer that had invaded my body. For months doctors took on the terrorist that lived within me. Together we fought with more than just my usually weapons and we were successful.

There were many steps taken together that made up the cancer war. All the steps that I took and that others took came together and saved my life.

In their hearts humans plan their course, but the Lord establishes their steps.

Proverbs 16:9

2.
LET'S ROLL

Todd Beamer boarded United Airlines Flight 93 on the morning of 9-11. He was traveling from the east coast to the west coast. The flight was disrupted when the passengers realized that the flight had been hijacked.

Todd Beamer was a former athlete at Wheaton College. His coaches said he was not only an athlete but also a Christian. He was a well-rounded young man who was very focused. Beamer had the characteristics of a solid leader.

No wonder Beamer took action on this flight. He was once an athlete on the baseball diamond and the basketball court, but now his field of play was in the sky. He gathered teammates and devised a plan. The team was not going to let their opponent crash into their conspired target.

Before they moved forward with their game plan, Beamer called an air phone supervisor. He informed her of what was happening in the air. He asked her if she would recite the Lord's Prayer with him and then asked if she would call his wife. When they finished the Lord's Prayer, Beamer set down the phone and was ready for the next play. The air phone operator listened. She heard Beamer say, "Are you guys ready? LET'S ROLL!"

32

In the locker room of the Wheaton College football team is the sign LET'S ROLL. As the players leave the locker room, they hit the sign. These two simple words have significant meaning.

These two words remind each player that they are part of a team. Each player is ready to go onto the field and execute the game plan. When the palm hits the metal, each team player is vowing to do their job. The touch of each palm says, "You can count on me." Each of their assignments may be different, but they all have a common goal.

The players know that it won't be easy. They will get hot, tired, and dirty, but it is all worth it.

Pregame

You, the patient, are now in the pregame. It is time for you to prepare to fight cancer. Preparation can be just as critical as the game itself. The pregame is going to fuel you physically, mentally, and spiritually. You will find information in these pages that were gathered from cancer patients and their teams. This information will guide you through your cancer journey.

To obtain as much information as I could, I began by going to those who could give me the best advice about cancer—cancer patients. Some I visited with, while others filled out a cancer patient survey that I had developed.

As I visited with cancer patients, hundreds of words began to roll off their tongues. The first question I asked was this:

What advice would you give someone who was diagnosed with cancer?

Listed below you will find the answers to that question. The cancer patients wanted you to know what they wished someone had told them in the beginning.

- God is bigger than any cancer.
- Attitude is everything, so stay positive.
- Always ask questions. No cancer question is unnecessary.
- Don't freak out when given a diagnosis. We found that the first thing you hear is usually the worst. Just have patience until all results are gathered
- Gather all information, explore options, discuss all treatment options with doctors and family, and pick the best treatment plan for you.
- Try to carry on life as normal.
- Cancer is not an automatic death sentence. Do not jump to conclusions.
- Let people help you. Whatever it is, accept the help and move on. It helps others when they can help you. Even let strangers help. They will become friends long after cancer has gone.
- If you are tired rest.
- Keep notes on everything, every doctor's appointment, every scan, every test.
- Keep a file containing all of your paperwork: scans, tests, insurance, bills, etc.
- Fight like hell.
- Do not Google anything.
- Find a doctor that you feel comfortable with.
- Make sure you have a good support system; if you don't have one, create one.
- People who have not experienced cancer may not say what you need to hear. Just move on. They don't get it.

- Pray more than you ever have.
- Believe in your doctors.
- Be thankful and grateful, for there is always someone worse than you.
- Be the germ police.
- Don't let the internet and others be your only advisors.
- Get a second opinion.
- Do not feel guilty about not being able to do what you used to do—this is temporary.
- Cry. It's ok—cancer is a scary thing.

It's not the will to win that matters—everyone has that. It's the will to prepare to win that matters.

Paul "Bear" Bryant

PERSONAL ESSAY

THE NEXT PLAY

J. B. Grimes
Tongue Cancer
Auburn Offensive Line Coach

"Frightened," that is how I felt. I have had several health issues through the years, but hearing the words "You have cancer" made me very anxious.

I was helmet to helmet with a giant, and I had to be a giant also. I followed what I have always believed in while coaching football. I devised a plan, set long term and short-term goals, and then began with baby steps. I understood the details and paid attention to them.

Tongue cancer was my diagnosis. It was detected very early. I was fortunate. Surgery was performed to remove part of my tongue and several lymph nodes located in my neck. I didn't have to go through any other treatment and within five days, with staples in my neck, I was back on the field with my players.

35

GO TO THE
NEXT PLAY
WHATEVER
THAT IS AND
DO YOUR BEST
NOT TO LOOK
AT THE
SCOREBOARD

Cancer is the opponent. How do we begin to devise a plan and set our goals? We understand this: opponents change; they have different schemes, but the fundamentals of the game stay the same.

One fundamental that is true is this: when you get knocked down, you get up. I was knocked down by cancer, but I didn't stay down long. Getting up and going wasn't smart on my part; however, staying as physically active as you can will do a lot for you mentally. Keeping a positive mindset isn't easy, but being positive always wins over negativity. Being positive is a choice, and it isn't easy waking up every day and choosing to be positive. Only you can control your attitude. When adversity strikes—and it will—go to the next play. In other words, keep fighting. I tell my players don't look at the scoreboard, just keep playing. With cancer, we should deal with it in the same way. Don't look at where you are. Look forward to the next play and keep playing.

Another fundamental is prayer. The Good Lord Himself told us, "Ask and you shall receive; knock and the door will be opened." Cancer is both mentally and physically tough. It has to be played by tough people. It takes God being placed in the center to increase your level of strength and endurance. The Lord will help in the day-to-day fight for what could be the battle of your life. Going through this has given me admiration for mentally tough people. The thing that makes it unique is they come in all different shapes and sizes.

The last fundamental is laughter. There is power behind laughing. At times it can be difficult, but try to laugh as much as you can. Laughter is the best medicine.

36

After Mass, I was thinking about my cancer journey, and the thought hit me. I have had five bypasses and four stents for a total of nine blockages in my heart. I have had cancer surgery. I have a bunch of scars located on my body. A wise man once told me, "A scar is proof that you beat whatever it was that tried to kill you. Wear them proudly."

A SCAR IS LIVING PROOF THAT YOU ARE A SURVIVOR.

PERSONAL ESSAY

THE PHONE CALL

Misti
Malignant Melanoma

Why is it that many times bad news is delivered through a phone call? I have had several phone calls over the years that stand out to me.

I have heard words on the other end of the line I didn't want to hear. Dad has cancer. Mom has cancer. YOU have cancer!

Cancer is something that has surrounded me for years. My dad was diagnosed with throat cancer then pancreatic cancer, my mom was diagnosed with colon cancer, and I was diagnosed with malignant melanoma. The word CANCER came through the phone receiver like it was being spoken over a loud speaker. The echo kept bouncing back and forth, even as I would try to shove it away. That word was not leaving.

It is at that moment when CANCER is spoken that you begin making a plan of action. What we found with all our diagnoses is that it takes time. Doctor appointments are made, and tests are scheduled.

37

In my situation, I had not one doctor but three—a dermatologist, a melanoma oncologist, and a plastic surgeon.

It was after I was given doctors' names and appointment times that I was placed in the holding pattern. I was in a stall waiting for the gate to be opened.

I was fortunate that my cancer was "in situ," meaning it was an early stage and the cancer was still confined to the site where it started. I had time to wait. My cancer was in one place and not going anywhere.

For some cancer patients, time is of the essence. You don't have time to wait. After the initial phone call, get going. Talk to your primary care physician. Ask them questions. Your PCP may be able to get an appointment for you quicker than you can. Get a cancer partner, someone you can count on to be a listening ear. As my husband says, "Everyone needs a heavy." A heavy is someone who will speak up, ask questions, and get the ball rolling.

Mine and my mother's phone calls were early; my dad's phone call was too late. Pick up the phone, devise a plan, gather your team, and get the ball rolling.

3.
THE TEAM

A team is a group of people who come together to achieve a common goal. You may be wondering why you need a team when you have cancer. Just like a competitive athletic team, every player comes to the field with a different set of skills required for an individual task. Everyone on your cancer team comes with different talents and strengths. You need every player with his or her different skills to create a win for your team.

You may have a large team, or you may have a small one. The size doesn't matter. All that matters is that everyone on the team has the same vision—to win.

Throughout these pages, you will find each person of your team defined and how that person functions as a significant part of your team. Every person is important. Teamwork enables common people to do uncommon things.

While our journey through the abyss of cancer could not have happened without holding tightly to our Lord Jesus, we want you to know that this book covers practical advice as well and serves as an inspiration for a deeper more meaningful life.

THE CANCER TEAM

HEAD COACH (Always on the field): GOD

HUDDLE: Patient (You are the ball. Everyone is handling you.) Doctors and caregiver (the star of the show)

CHEERLEADERS: Family or close friends

FANS: Those outside the circle who want to help

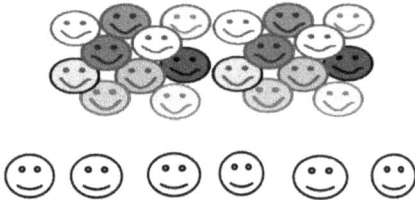

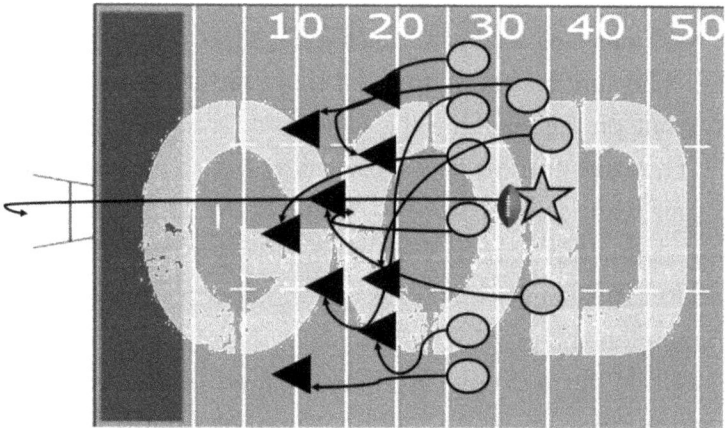

😊 Cheerleader
Family or Close Friends

🅑 FANS
Those outside the circle but
want to help

⬭ Your Team Huddle
Patient, Doctors and Caregivers

▶ Cancer (Visting Team)

⭐ Caregiver

🅞 You

OUR TEAM

Haley
Daughter

I have been on several teams during my lifetime, but I never dreamed our family would have to develop a cancer team. At 23, I was in the ordinary progression of my life, or at least I thought I was. I was in nursing school, had found the man I was marrying, and didn't have many worries, but then it happened.

As my dad was on a tractor, he began having seizures. He was rushed to the ER in our small community and then helicoptered to a bigger city. It was after several tests that the diagnosis of cancer was given to us. Astrocytoma stage 3.

Intrusive is all I can say about cancer. It invades the life of the patient and the patient's family. It disrupts the life of everyone.

When I thought of that day in April three years ago, I become nauseated. It makes me anxious, and I am reminded that cancer is the devil. Just as the devil causes chaos and confusion, cancer also does. It takes away life as we know it and forces everyone involved to find a new normal. Our new normal took a lot of people working together. We are very fortunate to have family in the same town, so everyone went to work. Our team started to form.

Tackling cancer takes many players. Everyone involved becomes your team. Doctors, surgeons, family, and friends each have a position to play. Everyone is in for the long haul no matter how many overtimes you have.

For just as each of us has one body with many members, and these members do not all have the same function, so in Christ we, though many, form one body, and each member belongs to all the others. We have different gifts, according to the grace given to each of us.

Romans 12:4–6a

As of today, we are going on three years, and we still have our team in place. Yes, some things have changed, but many of the people still have their position.

My dad has two friends who are devoted. The three of them have been friends since childhood. They come over sometimes every night of the week. They keep him up to date on what is going on in town; they bring him his favorites sweets and take him riding around the countryside. The most important thing they do is make him laugh. Laughter is the best medicine, and it takes his mind off of cancer.

We don't know how long our team will be in place, but no matter how long, our team will be glued together. Our whole team is committed. Everyone is important.

PERSONAL ESSAY
_____

HEADED FOR THE GOAL

Jackie
Caregiver

A cancer diagnosis is devastating on many different levels. It is not only difficult for the person with the diagnosis, but also for the caregiver and the immediate family.

My husband was a farmer who was on the farm all day working and talking to people about the ins and outs of agriculture. I worked for a medical facility an hour away from home. When he was diagnosed, our world completely changed. It wasn't something that happened gradually. He was on the farm, had a seizure, and that was it. The hammer hit us on the head. There was no time to spare.

42

When we first arrived at the hospital, they predicted several things—from a stroke to a tumor. Later the next day, they confirmed it was a tumor. Brain surgery was done. The surgery left my husband with no speech, very weak, and unable to do what everyday people do.

Since you now know part of my story, I want to go through some critical details.

First, I want to go back to the sentence *no time to spare*. When dealing with cancer, you have no time to waste. The medical system is cumbersome and very busy. Don't get lost in the system. If you are not familiar with the medical field, get someone who is to help you. Think of it as a ball game. You have the ball; you are the quarterback for your loved one. There is one minute left in the ballgame, and you must score. I have found, as the caregiver, that my job is to make sure the medical staff does what is necessary, in the correct and precise time, so that the score is made.

With cancer, you have to move toward the goal quickly. Don't underestimate the value of acting fast. You may need to seek out advice from others. It takes many teammates to make the team. Utilize anything and everything you can to find people who have had the same cancer. Even though all cancer diagnoses are different, they do have similarities. You may ask, how do I find others? In this day and time, social media can be a blessing; it can help you find people. I found a Facebook page of caregivers whose spouses have brain cancer. This social media was my first place to go and begin to ask questions.

Next, send someone to the store to get you a notebook with pockets. Keep everything; write down everything from day one. There are going to be times when you need to refer. I can't stress enough how important it is to write down everything from the time a medicine was taken, what kind of medicine was given, the names of doctors, the names of nurses, how much the patient ate, when they went to the bathroom, WHAT EACH DOCTOR SAID. You have to be aware and conscientious of every single thing. In this notebook, also write down questions you have. DON'T BE AFRAID TO ASK ANY AND EVERY QUESTION. You have the ball, and they are on your team. Since you only see your doctor now and then, you don't want to forget the questions you have.

Staying spiritually healthy is very important. Spirituality is what gives the foundation, desire, and momentum to seek physical health. I realized at first that I was praying only for healing. This wasn't exactly wrong, but it wasn't correct. Through this process, I realized I should be asking for strength, guidance, and clarity on navigating through this storm. Healing was going to come one way or another, but I was going to have to have the strength to handle whatever the healing was and how it was going to happen. It was God's plan, and it was good no matter what I wanted.

After things had got moving, my team had already started to form. My family, of course, were the ones to my rescue. They took over many things I couldn't physically do since I was with my husband an hour away from home. One thing to remember, though, is that you can't get your feelings hurt or get bitter. People will come and go through illnesses. Life goes on around cancer. While you are left treading water to keep from drowning, everyone else who isn't in the middle of the storm is doing the backstroke. Your team, like mine, will probably begin big and shrink in size over time.

Even though my team got smaller, I was very fortunate to have people who had knowledge in many areas of expertise. One of my childhood friends is in the insurance business. She immediately came to my rescue with answers to all bill and insurance questions. One of my brothers is a farmer, and one is a doctor, so they took care of many situations that I was left to handle without my husband. One of my daughters is a nurse, so she was a big help in helping take care of her dad. When you are placed in this situation, you can't be afraid to ask for help. If you need help call someone.

We are going on three years with brain cancer. Our scans are stable; we see miracles every day. Many are small, but they are still precious. Every day I read my bible, read my devotionals, and just keep on keeping on. We are headed to the goal one first down at a time.

IN SICKNESS AND HEALTH

Odes
Cancer Survivor and
Current Cancer Patient

Nancy
Caregiver, Teammate

Single and living in the city. I had met several people from work. Charlie Mae was one of them. Charlie Mae wanted me to meet her friend. Of course, I said I would. At church, her friend was standing next to the piano, but she wasn't standing alone. I walked over and introduced myself to the ladies. The next day Charlie Mae asked me if I wanted to take her friend on a date, I said, "No I liked the girl with her better." I hated to hear from Charlie Mae that she had a boyfriend and my dream date would not happen.

Soon after our first encounter, we all attended a gathering after church. The girl of my dreams, the one who stood by the piano wearing the hat, was there. Nancy was her name, and I wanted to go on a date with her. I decided I was going to ask her. I said, "Nancy if you weren't with Jim, I would ask you on a date." I was so surprised to learn that she wasn't with Jim and that she would go on a date with me. The rest is history. From then on, we have been partners for life.

We have not lived a life absent from adversity. We have had our share of ups and downs, but in the middle of the turmoil, I have always had peace. Worry free is how I have always been. John 14 has always carried me. I know that with Christ I have no troubles, and I know that my Father has a place for me in heaven. So why should I worry?

Cancer has knocked on my door several times along with some heart issues. I have survived ampullary cancer where the doctor performed the Whipple procedure. I had 18 inches of my colon removed because of colon cancer. I have had prostate cancer several times, and at present, it has returned.

Through all of this God, Nancy, and I have been partners. God put us together for a reason. When you look at people with entirely different backgrounds and different upbringings, you wonder how in the world they ended up together. But God knows. God knew we were the perfect match. I am the calm in Nancy's storm, and God is the calm in mine.

When faced with all my cancer diagnoses, Nancy and I looked for the best doctors. I asked questions. If I didn't ask the question, Nancy did. Nancy and I both educated ourselves about cancer. I now have many "ologists" as I call them. I believe in them. From my PCP, to my gastroenterologist, to my oncologists, they are all very good at what they do.

Nancy and I have taught Sunday school together, we have traveled together, we have raised kids together, we have enjoyed grandchildren together, and we have even ridden in an ambulance together. We have lived our lives together and fought cancer together.

We are partners, a team, that God put together at a church gathering in 1956. I meant it, and Nancy meant it—for better or worse, in sickness and health, until death do us part.

4.
THE COACH MATTERS

Dwight Adams was born in Arkansas in the 1930s. His mother decided she didn't want to be a mother. When he was five years old, she gave him away to the Arkansas Children's Home. There Adams lived as an orphan. He craved for a family. At one time, he hitch-hiked to where he knew his grandparents lived. He stood on their doorstep only to be told he was not wanted. The police escorted him back to the children's home.

It was in the children's home that the director, Ruth Beall, took particular interest in Dwight. She taught him many life lessons and offered him guidance. When he was in high school, his football coach, Wilson Matthews, knew there was something about this young man that was special. Wilson made sure he kept his eye on him.

Adams went on to play college ball and then began a career as a coach. He first coached high school and then advanced to college ball. He later went on to become involved in the NFL. Adams was the recruiter for the San Diego Chargers and finished his career as vice president of player personnel for the Buffalo Bills.

Adams was a larger-than-life gentle giant who gave credit to those where credit was due. He never forgot the two at the very beginning who believed in him and kept a thumb on him. He also credited all of the coaches who helped him along the way.

Coaches have a direct influence on the players in the game. Top-notch coaches produce winning players and teams. Coaches who maintain a positive attitude and create a positive environment end up with positive results. The relationship between the coach and players does matter.

Coaches made a direct impact on Dwight Adams's life. If it hadn't been for his high school coach Matthews, Adams might not have had as many life wins as he had. Matthew's influence developed him into the person and the coach he became. Adams valued the relationships he made with every player. He cherished the game, but more than that he treasured the life lessons he could share with the players he felt were his own. Adams was a coach at heart. That is probably why everyone called him "COACH!"

COACH: ONE WHO INSTRUCTS AND TRAINS, ONE WHO TEACHES IN THE FUNDAMENTALS AND DIRECTS TEAM STRATEGY.

God Is Our Coach

Just like a coach has a direct influence on his or her players, God has a direct impact on you as the patient. God is the coach at the center of the game. He knows the plays, calls the plays, and finalizes the plays.

The relationship between you and God is the most important. It is the relationship with Him that gives you hope. Trusting in Him while battling in a game that has very few answers can be difficult. What you must do is fix your eyes on God and his promises.

God never promised anyone that life would be easy or that life would be without hardships. God is

49

always working in the midst of what seems senseless. You will never understand the why of cancer, and even if you did, you probably wouldn't be satisfied with the answer. Knowing the why wouldn't change the situation. You only need to understand that the "how" is more important. How are you going to get through this? Many cancer patients know the answer to that question. Faith helps you get through cancer. God works together for your good. Things work out, lessons are learned, and everyone involved grows in wisdom. Even in the darkness, God gives you the hope you need to find the purpose and the joy.

A friend once told me this: In some situations, education doesn't matter. It is the experience that counts.

When experiencing something like cancer, it is through you that God can be glorified. God wants you to use your experiences to share with others the good work He can do. Sharing your stories to help others is the purpose of the pain.

God is your coach He is the head coach. He is the one you should go to first for advice. He knows the plays, and He knows the plan. He will instruct you on the fundamentals and devise the strategies that will be helpful. He knows.

ONLY THE HEAD COACH IS INVITED

At the beginning of the list created by cancer patients are the words GOD IS BIGGER THAN CANCER. God is bigger than everything, and He doesn't invite cancer into your life. Cancer, our enemy, is not invited; it simply shows up.

Envision this: You are a huge fan of the Razorbacks. Every item you have on from your hat to your shoes is red. You are even wearing a Razorback hog nose. You get your popcorn and your coke and sit in your seat ready for the game. You notice that many of the seats around you are not filled. The game is about to begin when you see that the opposing team's fans are filling the empty seats around you. There is no more red in sight. Purple has taken over your cheering section.

I know we are supposed to love our enemies, but how would you feel? How would you feel if you were ready to cheer on your favorite team and you were shut down by the opposing fans? The enemy, the opposition, took a seat right next to you!

This is how cancer is; it invites itself to take a seat right next to you. Cancer decides to show up in your cheering section. Cancer is the opponent that arrives for the game thinking that it is going to overtake you. Cancer tries to walk into your stands and make itself at home, but the key word here is TRIES.

When diagnosed with cancer, one of the first questions is "Why? I didn't invite cancer to take a seat in my body. Why did this happen to me?"

At times, we have the answer to the why, but on other occasions, there is no rhyme or reason for it to show up.

I began to ask the question "What part does God play in cancer?" In Lysa Terkeurst's book *Uninvited*, I found the perfect answer nestled within her words:

> The world is in a state of decay and corruption. We see it in deadly weather patterns, natural disasters, and famines that were not part of God's good design. Cancer, sickness, and disease ARE

A coach will impact more young people in a year than the average person does in a lifetime.

Billy Graham

I will instruct you and teach you in the way you should go; I will counsel you with my loving eye on you.

Psalm 32:8

NOT PART OF GOD'S GOOD DESIGN. Car accidents, drownings, and murders were not part of God's good design.

BAD THINGS WERE NOT PART OF GOD'S PLAN. You can go back and blame Adam and Eve and Satan for cancer. When Adam and Eve were enjoying the beautiful garden, Satan decided to invite himself. He didn't need an invitation. He just showed up with his crafty, beautiful self. Of course, being an excellent hostess, Eve didn't want to be rude, so what did she do? She began listening to Satan. In her mind, she questioned, "Did God really tell me not to eat from the tree?" Satan was compelling, and of course, Eve fell into Satan's trap of lies. The minute Adam and Eve touched their lips to the brilliant shining piece of fruit, it happened. Sin was invited into the world. Satan took full advantage. He not only worked through sight but also through thoughts.

At that point, Satan grinned and God cried!

Cancer invites itself into the body and Satan takes full advantage of the invitation. Satan tries to convince us that God doesn't love us or that He is punishing us. Satan works diligently placing thoughts between our ears. He loves it when he brings feelings of anxiety, fear, and hopelessness into our bodies.

In the book *The Spirit of Python*, Jentezen Franklin gives a fabulous analogy of Satan. He compares Satan to that of a python. A python's job is to grab its prey, encircle it, and tighten its grip. Then it squeezes the breath out of its victim until there is no breath left.

Be aware of Satan. He is going to try to work this cancer diagnosis until he can squeeze the breath out of you. BUT you are not going to let that happen. You are not going to give Satan the opportunity to take captive your thoughts. You are NOT going to become bitter or hopeless. You are not going to let him take you down in a headlock. You have protection!

So, with all of that being said, we know that from the moment sin entered the world the human race would endure hardships. How can we be certain of this? The Bible tells us so!

> *Consider it pure joy, my brothers and sisters, whenever you face trials of many kinds, because you know that the testing of your faith produces perseverance. Let perseverance finish its work so that you may be mature and complete, not lacking anything. If any of you lacks wisdom, you should ask God, who gives generously to all without finding fault, and it will be given to you. But when you ask, you must believe and not doubt, because the one who doubts is like a wave of the sea, blown and tossed by the wind. That person should not expect to receive anything from the Lord. Such a person is double-minded and unstable in all they do.*
> James 1:2-8

So take note: if you are blaming God, don't. You need Him. You need Him more now than you ever have. God doesn't invite cancer into our bodies. He suffers when He sees us suffer. God cries when He sees us cry. He doesn't want His children to go through hardships. He is not a God of chaos and confusion. He is a God of peace and patience.

Even through cancer, God wants the best for you. There are instances God may allow cancer to happen, but it isn't because of your sin or because of your parents' sin. It is simply part of God's bigger plan for your life. His plans are best even when you don't

Leadership, like coaching, is fighting for the hearts and souls of men and getting them to believe in you.

Eddie Robinson

God answers prayers, but he doesn't always answer it your way.

Lou Holtz

understand. At times cancer may just be like a thorn in your flesh.

When you face your fiercest opponent, God is there. He walks on the field with you as you put on your armor and go for the goal. Sometimes cancer is allowed so that God can shine through you. He can show up and show out! God wants you to use your cancer experiences so that others can see His glory.

> *Finally, be strong in the Lord and in his mighty power. Put on the full armor of God, so that you can take your stand against the devil's schemes. For our struggle is not against flesh and blood, but against the rulers, against the authorities, against the powers of this dark world and against the spiritual forces of evil in the heavenly realms. Therefore put on the full armor of God, so that when the day of evil comes, you may be able to stand your ground, and after you have done everything, to stand. Stand firm then, with the belt of truth buckled around your waist, with the breastplate of righteousness in place, and with your feet fitted with the readiness that comes from the gospel of peace. In addition to all this, take up the shield of faith, with which you can extinguish all the flaming arrows of the evil one. Take the helmet of salvation and the sword of the Spirit, which is the word of God. And pray in the Spirit on all occasions with all kinds of prayers and requests. With this in mind, be alert and always keep on praying for all the Lord's people.*
> Ephesians 6:10-18

God sits with you just as He sat with the disciples. Don't start questioning and doubting. I know what you think, because all of us doubt. You may be saying, "I have sinned. Why would God want to help me through this? Why would He want to help me uninvite this cancer?"

54

Let me tell you right now, stop doubting. YOU ARE FALLING INTO SATAN'S TRAP. When you are in the locker room, get rid of Satan's voice between your ears. Only listen to the One who loves you. God is love. He loves you no matter what sin you have committed. Before you step onto the field of play, go to Him. Tell Him you are here and you want Him on this journey with you. Tell Him that you cannot do this without Him. He already knows this, but He is just waiting for the invitation to walk with you.

For God is not a God of disorder but of peace—as in all the congregations of the Lord's people.

1 Corinthians 14:33

If you have children, you will know what I mean when I say God has a love of a parent for a child. You are God's child. HE LOVES YOU! He wants to fight this fight with you. He wants to be in the game of life with you. He wants to coach you and cheer for you. You are never alone because He is with you.

As Jesus sat with His disciples for the last moments, He told them many important things. The last thing that he told them in John 16 was this:

I have told you these things, so that in me you may have peace. In this world, YOU WILL HAVE TROUBLE. But take heart! I have overcome the world.

John 16:33

As Joel Osteen explained in his lesson "Don't Waste Your Pain," he speaks of adversity and how to use the trouble that we do have in this world.

Satan turns on the heat, but God controls the thermostat. Satan had to ask God to test Job. God told him he could test him, but not take his life. God knows what we can handle. It is through these times that God wants us to learn and use it to glorify Him. It is difficult to understand, but when we deal with situations of bad, we need to see it as a gift. With the pain, we are being devel-

"For I know the plans I have for you," declares the Lord, "plans to prosper you and not to harm you, plans to give you hope and a future."

Jeremiah 29:11

oped to reach the fullness of our destiny. There is a purpose for the pain and that purpose is to help us grow so that later we can be instrumental in helping others overcome. This pain leads to gain.

You will have trouble, things will take a seat in your life that you don't invite, you will have thorns in your flesh, you will face fierce opponents, BUT you will have peace because you are safe holding Jesus's hand on your field of play. The Lord is your head coach and He is calling all the plays.

Cancer may have taken a seat in your cheering section, but with God, you can kick him out of the game.

Personal Essay

Practice What You Preach

Dr. John Sullivan
Bladder and Colon Cancer

The diagnosis was traumatic. The word cancer landed upon my ears. Located in the bladder and the colon was the cancer. Removal of the bladder was the first decision that was made for my survival. The doctor's decision may have been removal of the bladder, but my decision was faith and prayer.

It was then that I was going to have to practice what I have preached all these years—just have faith and pray without ceasing. Through seven surgeries and years of fighting, Jesus was with me. Without Him, I would have quit trying, but I knew He was walking this fight right beside me.

God is with us during the trials of life. James 1:1-4 tells us to consider it pure joy whenever we face trials because the testing of our faith produces perseverance. The pure joy is not in the trial itself but the outcome. I look back over the years with cancer and realize that I am a better person. I am better, not bitter. I have stayed close to the Lord.

Many times, when people have been going through adversity, I have been asked why? Why did this happen to me? Why did this happen to my family? There is no question or answer to the why. The only question we should have is what? What does this adversity allow me to learn about my Lord, my faith, and myself?

One of the greatest lessons, when given a diagnosis of cancer, is that God is in control. Whether the doctor gives us a temporary diagnosis or a terminal diagnosis, God is the keeper of the answer. Ephesians 2:10-12 explains to us that we are God's masterpiece. Because of this, we must understand that God is in control of our salvation. It is his powerful work in us that makes us his work of art. We should treat ourselves with respect taking care of our physical bodies and realizing that God is the hope we have to press forward. He can take our unclean condition and make us pure.

> For God so loved the world that he gave his one and only Son, that whoever believes in him shall not perish but have eternal life.
>
> John 3:16

God loves us. He gave his son to die on a cross for us. By believing in Him and leaning on faith, a person will realize that even if given a terminal diagnosis, they will have eternal life with God.

I have learned to live with cancer as long as God allows. My joy has increased not in the trial but the

Be strong and courageous. Do not be afraid or terrified because of them, for the Lord your God goes with you; he will never leave you nor forsake you."

Deuteronomy 31:6

Therefore, in order to keep me from becoming conceited, I was given a thorn in my flesh, a messenger of Satan, to torment me.

2 Corinthians 12:7

journey and the outcome. Jesus loves me through it all. Trusting in Him is the only thing that matters.

I am in remission now, but you never know when it will return. I keep preaching faith, hope, trust, and patience. I keep praying, and others keep praying for me also.

My doctor was able to save my bladder. I thanked him. He replied by saying, "It is probably due to the many who have been praying for you."

Lesson learned: **Practice what you preach!**

THE CHOICE

Amy
Breast Cancer Survivor

There was NO OTHER CHOICE but to survive. Being 38 and having two children, ages three and eight, there was no option for me. I was going to win. I wasn't going to fold physically or mentally. I knew I was going to get through it, and I knew what the outcome was going to be.

With cancer, there are many different things to consider. It is critical that you are in the right hands. Doctors begin throwing things out at you, but ultimately you get to decide. From the very beginning, I decided I was going to make the best decision to get the best results no matter what I had to do. I had made the choice I was going to have a mastectomy. One doctor thought a mastectomy wasn't necessary. My other doctor asked me, "What do you want to do?" I replied "Mastectomy." He said, "Good. That is what I think you should do." This was part one of me doing what I had to do for survival.

It has been 14 years since my diagnosis with breast cancer, so some things aren't as fresh on my mind. I do remember, however, that I made the decision and was going to give it my best shot. I'm sure there was some fear, but I don't remember being fearful. Fear didn't consume me because it was the first time I felt the love of the Lord.

I had a love relationship with Him, and He was going to get me through this. I was in constant conversation with Christ. He led me through every step. Not only was God's love evident, but also how others showed love was prevalent. There has never been another time when I have seen an overabundant amount of love from my friends and even from complete strangers. If there is something good from cancer this is it—LOVE.

I have never looked back or had a fear of the cancer reoccurring. Cancer doesn't make you an automatic candidate for death. None of us are guaranteed tomorrow even if we are healthy.

Being goal oriented, I set my goal at the beginning of my cancer diagnosis. My goal was to watch my babies grow up. I didn't give cancer the choice to define my life and rob me of the days ahead. I made the decision with God to survive, and that is what I have done.

My children are now 21 and 17. We don't revisit my cancer. It is in the past. I don't live worrying it may return; I live each day pressing forward to tomorrow. My choice is to live.

But seek first his kingdom and his righteousness, and all these things will be given to you as well.

Matthew 6:33

BROKEN

Sarah
Breast Cancer

The brokenness IS the beauty.

Father, show me what the enemy doesn't want me to see. Again and again as of late, this has been the prayer of my heart. I'm sick and tired of feeling STUCK. Of feeling as if I've lived the same day for almost two years now. A stuck so deep that there are rarely even words. Just tears. And groans. And fetal positions.

And can I just be honest, for the love? This past year has been THE hardest of my 38 to date. I thought the year after the diagnosis—surely that was the pinnacle of pain. Turns out, not so much. The mental, emotional, and spiritual game have been strong in year two. Much more so than I could have EVER imagined. And almost two years in, the battle rages. For those of you who wonder, Yes, I'm still contending for my physical healing. Couple that with the exhaustive mental and emotional toll that "fighting for your life" takes nearly every waking second of every day, and is it any wonder that bedtime is my favorite time? Because at least in my sleep, I can forget. Or maybe it's surrender. A trusting in God that I WILL, in fact, wake up again tomorrow and live to see another day. Hum. I can trust Him with my sleeping hours but still feel such a need to control my waking hours. As if the responsibility to stay alive is somehow mine. Ugh. The weight of it. I know. YES. I know. It's delusional. And it's NOT the truth. It's a straight up LIE. But one that my actions would say I have believed. Even though I

KNOW and have known from the beginning that the HEALING is NOT—I repeat is NOT—MY job.

So yeah, broken. That's the one word I can find to somehow depict the way I feel on the inside. Just. Broken. Like in a bazillion fractured pieces. So unrecognizably broken that I wonder sometimes if the pieces of ME will EVER fit again. And if I'll be as disfigured on the inside as I am on the outside. Is there any hope AFTER the brokenness, I wonder?

And so this morning, as I walk this stretch of pristine perfection, soaking in all that my senses can take in, I pray that prayer again—"Lord, show me what the enemy doesn't want me to see." And in the very next step, the sand changed. The fluffy, soft white sand gave way to a small stretch of coarser sand, and my feet felt, and my eyes saw, and my mind remembered what I'd just read the night before about how these waters are some of the brightest, vibrant shades of turquoise the eyes have ever seen. And just like that, the scales fell from my eyes, and I SAW.

The brokenness.

The brokenness IS the beauty.

Turks and Caicos boast some of the most beautiful beaches in the world. With water so stunningly clear blue that people often wonder if the pics have been filtered up and Photoshopped. I assure you—the answer is no. Creation does not disappoint. For the record, the Creator doesn't either. But that's a post for another day. And a truth I sometimes maybe still forget.

So, this blue. This breathtaking blue. Of all the colors we can and do see in the ocean, is it not this bright light turquoise that we find ourselves mesmerized by? Enamored by? C'mon, above the deep dark blue and the greens, isn't turquoise your fave? Isn't that what we flock to?

Last night as I read online about the local beaches and the abundance of turquoise water, I came to know WHY. Gosh—y'all know I'm a WHY girl :). It turns out, most of the T&C Islands are surrounded by a coral reef, thus providing the islands some natural protection. The sand I read about, like most sand, is made from the BREAKING down of coral and seashells. And THIS. This is what my feet felt, and my mind remembered, and my heart begins to grasp.

The brokenness IS the beauty.

The BREAKING of what WAS gives way to what WILL BE. And though we may EVOLVE, NOTHING ever really dies. Not REALLY. Not in the big picture. Not in His picture. And I keep on keeping on—one foot in front of the other. Processing how this beautiful beach that I love so much—that WE love so much, that we marvel at and travel insane distances to seek out—this sandy stretch where two worlds collide is actually that. Where two purposes collide. Yeah. This beautiful thing IS the brokenness. And this whole ocean...the shore...I watch every detail. The waves, the rocks, the fish, the marine plants. Everything is brimming with LIFE. And NONE of it is striving. None of God's OTHER creations work for their role. They all just seem to know how to BE. To be WHO they were made to be. To literally roll with the tide. And I am slightly jealous. Okay, no. Highly jealous.

And I step into the blue. The bright turquoise that whispers "Come and BE refreshed. BE renewed. Come and soak in Me." And I do. And I finally lower my hands to the water. And in it, I am aware of my otherwise normal posture with hands often clenched and drawn inward. Always concealing. Always protecting. Always defending. Always ready to fight back. And this has been my way for the past two years, probably much longer if we're honest. Fight or flight. And yeah, I am WEARY. Rest and Receive. Rest and Receive. Rest and Receive. Aren't these the first of words the Lord would utter to me after diagnosis. Rest. And Receive.

Ah. How long does it take this stubborn one to grasp Your truths, Lord? How. Stinking. Long.

Oh, the blue. I set my hands upon the water and gaze out upon the vastness. And then my eyes find their way down. That fluffy soft white sand beneath my feet. Water at my chest but so clear I can see every ridge in the sand and scar on my feet...and I remember WHY the turquoise is turquoise. It's because of the sand below. The sand that through the nature of a rugged life—through wave after wave, beating after beating, coral and shell that were crushed and pressed into something NEW. And here's the REAL beauty...that hue that we all love. That blue that takes our breath away. It IS what it is because of the light reflecting off the water and the brokenness that lies beneath.

The light. Oh. The Light.

As Ann Voskamp's book *The Broken Way* reminds us, maybe the broken places let the light get in better.

And maybe it's not the dark blues of our deep blessings or the greens of our growth but the turquoise of our troubles that BEST lets the light in. That best let the Sun shine through. Maybe there IS something to living the Broken Way. Maybe there IS something to owning the hard, to feel our feelings, to shed our tears and groan when the pain is just too unspeakable. Maybe. Just maybe. The REAL beauty. The kind that draws the eye and heart toward the One who made and loves us beyond understanding…MAYBE He doesn't want me JUST when I'm happy and blessed and growing. But when I'm lamenting, crying, and groaning too. MAYBE it's in THAT place. In the middle of my messy. My ugly. My hard. My absolute shattered brokenness that God can do His MOST BEAUTIFUL work. Maybe it's the (Son) LIGHT that CAPTURES the beauty. That reframes the Broken and lets us REALLY see. Maybe it's OUR brokenness that reflects HIS brokenness. And if His was beautiful and for a purpose greater than Himself, MAYBE mine is too.

Maybe.

Just. Maybe

Friends. If you too have been silent in your broken, be encouraged. He SEES you. And more than that, He longs to shine SO brightly in it and through it. He longs to turn what feels like sharp, rugged rubble into a masterpiece SO breathtaking, the world marvels. And all glory is HIS. Let Him shine in your broken, my friend.

LET.

HIM.

SHINE.

No more faking "fine."

This IS the Broken Way.

And in the Broken, there is Beauty.

5.
THE MENTAL MINDSET

You are probably going to have a short period where you feel defeated after receiving a diagnosis, but just as Lou Holtz said after his house burned, "The good Lord put eyes in the front of your head and not the back for a reason. We will have an amount of time to feel bad for ourselves and then move forward."

Lou Holtz was a very positive Christian coach. He said, "I never had a player not fall down. However, the great players always get up. It is all about the attitude. We have a choice whether we are going to get up or stay down. The most important piece is to believe you are going to win. Never let the opposition think you aren't in control. Refuse to lose."

When Holtz coached at Arkansas, they were facing a dangerous opponent. Arkansas was expected to lose. When he gave the locker room speech, however, he continually told the players, "When the press asks you how you won, tell them we were the better team." He never spoke as if they were going to lose; he said to them—"when we win."

When we step on the playing field, we must not only be prepared physically but also mentally. Developing our mental mindset enhances our performance and determines our success. Decide that your attitude is going to be a winning one.

Choose not to lose.

Cancer can be mentally grueling, demanding, and intense. All of your thoughts can either give peace to your soul or send your soul into a state of turmoil.

It is imperative that during the pregame you get control of your mind and learn how to focus and refocus. Being able to focus allows you to perform your best and prevents you from being distracted.

When I asked a therapist, Amanda Norcross, to explain the importance of mental health while going through cancer, she listed several important factors:

- Remember that all the emotions you are feeling are normal. You might feel anger, grief, fear, hope, all of the above, something else, or a confusing mixture of emotions you can't even name at first. This is to be expected; it is your body and mind doing their job, alerting you to what you need. Our emotions convey messages that can help us know what to do when we take the time to listen. For example, anger might mean you need to speak up in some way or to act on your behalf regarding your treatment; grief probably means there are losses to be mourned; fear might mean you need to reach out for support.

- Make space for and attend to the emotions you are experiencing. It might seem paradoxical, but allowing space for your emotions increases both your physical and emotional health. It keeps your body and mind from holding the extra tension of pent-up feelings and reduces your emotional brit-

tleness. Emotions are not meant to be kept in—
they are intended to move through us, like a wave.
In fact, the word "emotion" comes from the Latin,
"*emovere*," which means to move through. And all
emotions do move through. It can feel as if they
will last forever, but they rise and then naturally
lessen. When you can allow this, your body and
mind will be more resilient.

- Stay connected with other people as much as you
  can. You need to be able to turn inward to process
  what is happening internally, and you might just
  need to be alone sometimes. You also need to have
  at least one person who offers you reliable
  support—someone who feels soothing, reassuring,
  encouraging, or someone who understands your
  situation. Our bodies and brains are deeply wired
  to be in relationships with others and seek comfort
  from others. Without that connection, we experience much higher levels of physical and emotional distress.

- Consider seeking out psychotherapy. Therapy can
  be a highly valuable part of your care because it
  both provides support in sorting through your
  emotions and gives you connection with others.
  You can meet with a therapist one-on-one, you
  can join a therapy group with others who are also
  going through cancer, or you might find some
  other method of treatment that works for you.
  Whatever approach you choose, your therapy
  experience should help you feel less alone and
  more understood. Asking for therapist recommendations from your doctors, other patients, or

friends can help you find someone who seems like a good fit for you. And while you might have support from family and friends, therapy can be a valuable addition to your treatment because it provides you with a safe space where you can adequately express what you are experiencing without having to worry about upsetting or overwhelming your loved ones.

- Remember that emotions from the past might be mixed with the present. You might find that unresolved or unfelt emotions from previous experiences emerge during your diagnosis and treatment. Perhaps a loved one died when you were young, or you were taught that needing help is weak, or emotional upset wasn't allowed in your family. Such experiences can complicate your current emotional experience and your treatment. If you feel as though your past and present are getting mixed up in this way, working with a therapist can help. A therapist can help you not just understand your current emotional response better but also help lay those past experiences to rest.

- Be intentional about self-care. Doing kind things for yourself can provide islands of soothing and a sense of being able to do something important for yourself in the midst of what can be an overwhelming, out-of-control-feeling experience. Even if it is something that seems small, taking the time to do things for yourself that feel comforting can make a big difference in how you feel emotionally. Find what feels good to you—maybe take a bath, make yourself a cup of tea, read things that make you feel good, wear comfy pajamas, or spend a few minutes outside. And if you find it hard to make this happen, it can help so much to practice being kind to yourself.

- Caregivers need support, too. Those who are walking with you through your diagnosis and treatment—partners, parents, children—also need space and time to attend to their emotions and feel support from others. All of the recommendations here apply to them as well.

Your mind directly impacts how well you play. None of us want to lose so we must believe in our team. You must be prepared to deliver your A+ performance. To achieve this, you must be certain that your enemy doesn't dwell in your mind.

HOW TO STAY MENTALLY ON TOP OF YOUR GAME

- SEEK GOD FIRST (Pray, meditate, breathe— these will calm the nerves.)

- VISUALIZE YOURSELF HEALTHY (Find a picture of you when you look great and post it on your mirror.)

- CONTROL THE CONTROLLABLE (Serenity prayer. You are in control of your thoughts. Change the negative into positive.)

- REST (It is okay to be tired and say no to things that used to be normal.)

The five S's of sports training are: stamina, speed, strength, skill, and spirit; but the greatest of these is spirit.

Ken Doherty

- POSITIVE TALK (Find your positive quote and live by it. Use it to refocus when thinking negatively. Gather key phrases, words, songs anything to keep you positive. This could be a fight song. See a therapist who will help you understand that how you are feeling is normal.)

- BELIEVE YOU ARE A WINNER (You can achieve the challenge in front of you.)

- JOURNAL (Writing down your thoughts and feelings will allow you to let go of tension and anxiety. Write it down and then let it go. Express feelings that you have.)

- LIVE FOR TODAY (Do not spend time worrying about yesterday or tomorrow.)

- ROUTINE (Try to keep things as normal as possible. Begin a cancer routine. How you spend time the night before and the day of treatments will lessen your anxiety if you prepare before and create a routine.)

- TAKE CARE OF YOU (Do things that make you feel good, things that will boost your spirits. Plan outings with friends. Don't isolate yourself.)

This takes time to master, but practice makes perfect. You will have to experiment and see what works for you. You may rather do five than 10. It is your choice. This is something you can control—how you choose to control your brain. Develop your desired mindset and practice. It will begin to click, and your performance will be able to win any challenge that is placed ahead of you.

Staying positive can be difficult when you have the weight of cancer pressing down on you. Listed below are some of the answers given by cancer patients on how to stay mentally on top of your game:

- Rely on God—have a big faith.
- Cling to God's promises.
- Never let cancer dominate you emotionally or spiritually.
- Realize you have a lot to live for—family, grandkids, etc.
- Find blessings in everything.
- Find something every day you are thankful for.
- Pray.
- Laugh at yourself.
- Continue to work.
- Go about your everyday life as normal as possible.
- Meditate.
- Read the Bible.
- Journal.
- Rely on your church family.
- Keep a winning attitude. Never doubt you will win.
- Read daily journal.
- Find quotes that make you mentally stronger.
- Surround yourself with a positive group of people.
- Cry if you need to.
- Remember that everyone has something they are dealing with. Yours just happens to be cancer.
- Try to be an inspiration to others who are also dealing with a giant.
- Talk honestly about the situation.
- Focus on anything and everything that brings happiness.

ATTITUDE IS EVERYTHING, AND A WINNING ATTITUDE IS MORE THAN EVERYTHING.

Above all else, guard your heart, for everything you do flows from it.

Proverbs 4:23

- Exercise when you feel like it.
- Give hugs!
- It is okay to take anti-anxiety medicine. This doesn't make you a weak person.

PERSONAL ESSAY

MONSTER MOTIVATOR

Misti
Mom, Cheerleader

Kirk
Doctor

Sarah
Breast Cancer Warrior

Monsters are scary creatures. They bring fear and distraction. The funny thing is they are imaginary. They are not real, but we let monster thoughts take over.

While visiting with my brother-in-law who is a physician, I asked his thoughts on cancer. One thing that stood out during our visit was this: "Two people can have the same diagnosis, the same staging, the same treatment, and end up with different outcomes because they took two different pathways. A patient can take the path of hell or the path of inspiration."

Two years before his diagnosis, our son-in-law began studying the mental aspect of the athlete. I know that this was the Lord preparing him for what was ahead. The psychological piece to cancer is of most importance. Not just in cancer, but in life. Over 70,000 thoughts go off in our head every day. Those ideas can be monster or Godly. We have to learn how

72

to control our thoughts. We have to focus on Godly thoughts that speak the truth versus monster thoughts that speak inaccuracy.

Our friend Sarah, who has been battling breast cancer for several years quoted impressive true statements about thoughts:

Make sure your worst enemy doesn't live between your own two ears.

Laird Hamilton

> Lies flood in our mind thousands of times per day. To me, that is a whole lot of stinking thinking that leads us to a pit of destruction. It takes intense focus to take every monster thought captive and intentionally change it to a Godly thought. We have to wrestle in opposition to contend with the enemy for control over our mind. When we look at the word "contend," it means to wrestle in opposition, to contend with the enemy for control of the port. The port is where someone or something comes in and out. Our port is our mind where our thoughts come in and out. We have a battle going on between our ears at all times. Our thoughts shape words, words become actions, actions become habits, habits become our lives, and so thoughts become our lives. We have to take the port captive and get rid of the negative thoughts. Reject the lies and replace with the truth. We must recognize to reconcile. We have to mind our mind. It is not the thing that holds us back. It is how we think about the thing that harbors us. We may not be able to control what comes into our port, but we can choose what stays and what we kick to the curb. We can give our thoughts power through our words. Don't speak your thoughts and give them power. Marinate on the good and speak peace into the internal waves. God is in control of the wind and the waves. It isn't our circumstances that take us out. It is what we think about our circumstances that gets us. If we think it, we speak it, and then we give life to it. Don't give life to the negative thoughts. Take

charge of your internal atmosphere. Overcome and take your thoughts captive. What do you want your outcome to be? If you want your outcome to be one of peace, then begin today taking captive the monster thoughts that linger in and out of your port.

On your team, you will have the MVPs, the cheerleaders, the fans, and the other teammates, but the bottom line is you have to master becoming your mind motivator. You can call everyone into the huddle to be positive, but you still have to believe it yourself. You have to take control of your port.

Don't let the scary, fearful monster thoughts destroy your mind. Let monster motivating Godly thoughts penetrate your soul and bring you peace. When you focus on His thoughts, your port will be powered by His voice.

PERSONAL ESSAY

Don't Freak Out
Kathleen
Ovarian Cancer Patient

I'm sure you are reading this and thinking to yourself, "Sure, don't freak out!" This was the first thing I said to my husband (but not necessarily what I said to myself). I then went on to say under my breath like a friend of mine when she told her mom she had a tattoo, "I have a mass." Her mom couldn't hear very well, but she did hear the word tattoo, just as my husband heard the word mass. He didn't freak out, but he did go into silent mode. He soon snapped out of it when he learned we were headed to the oncologist the next day and our appointment was at 6:45 a.m.

On the way over, I thought about the mass that made me look like a pregnant woman carrying a seven-pound baby. At the age of 50, I didn't think it was amusing, but my 30-year-old son, before we knew it was cancer, thought it was hilarious. The only thing I wanted "mass" to mean was the Mass service I attend every week at our Catholic church.

When we arrived at Carti, I was greeted by wonderful sweet people who had me sign many papers and then took my blood. I then met with the doctor who called me princess and gave me a hug. So far everything was going well, no freak out for me yet. He explained that from the look of my scan, the mass did present itself as cancer. However, he needed to drain the fluid to see what we were dealing with. Off I went to outpatient to have my pregnant looking stomach removed. They drained 8 pounds 4 ounces of fluid. No wonder my son teased me; the fluid was bigger than he was at birth.

I was to call the doctor back to find out the results. Once again, in one of those quiet tattoo voices, I heard the doctor on the other end confirm the results, "Yes, it is cancer."

I still didn't freak out. Many of my friends did, though. I have learned some people are just more dramatic than I am. Some freak out and some don't. From day one I had decided that I was going to be strong as a rock and hold it together. Not that I don't have a few crumbling days, but that is why we have glue. I carry my glue with me to stick me back together. How can I freak out when I have wonderful doctors and supportive friends and family?

Set your minds on things above, not on earthly things.

Colossians 3:2

I am three years in and still doing chemo. I still haven't had a bad freak-out moment. I have learned when I feel a moment coming on I just say, "I trust you, Jesus." This has helped me see God in every situation. This strategy works, and it keeps me from freaking and being stressed.

Being mentally positive during cancer is as important as treatment. I feel that your mental state is directly related to your physical outcome. It does the body no good to had extra stress.

PERSONAL ESSAY

CHANGE FOR THE POSITIVE

Kerry
Caregiver

I had no other option but to be positive. My husband was diagnosed with stage 3A lung cancer. He didn't want anyone to know. CANCER was his diagnosis, and he was going to fight it. Our team consisted of my husband and me.

Since I couldn't let anyone in on our secret, I had to find a way for both of us to survive. The devil was trying to take us out, but God was not going to allow that. He was going to build our faith. My only option was to pray without ceasing and change every negative to a positive.

Before my husband began his treatment, the doctor gave us the dreaded list of what could happen, otherwise called "the list of what to expect." This is where the positive came into play. On a piece of paper, I made two columns. One column was for the negative and one was for the positive. With every negative side effect, I listed a positive. I prayed against the negative and prayed FOR THE POSITIVE.

KEEP CALM AND CARRY ON! DON'T FREAK OUT!

NEGATIVE	POSITIVE
Tired	Not tried
Unable to work	Won't miss work
Sick	Will not be sick

During treatments, I never missed one of my prayer sessions praying for the positive. My husband drove himself to every treatment, never missed a day of work, wasn't overly tired, and was not sick. The only side effect that he had was hair loss, and we could deal with that.

Prayer works. God is a powerful and great physician.

PERSONAL ESSAY

Psycho!

Cancer Wife

Cancer can show up in any lymph node in our body. In a patient who has had no detection of cancer, a lymph node that has grown from .3mm to .8mm would probably not be alarming. However, in a cancer patient, everything is noticed.

So here we go. A CT scan is performed that shows a few lymph nodes have grown in size. The doctor calls and says, "We don't want to alarm you, but my nurse is going to be calling you with an appointment for a PET scan. You have a few lymph nodes that look funny."

ALARM YOU! What do you think? Of course, this is going to ALARM ME! Then you tell me that the radiologists are PSYCHO! BUT DON'T WE WANT THEM TO BE? Of course, we do. When you mix a radiologist's report, a doctor's call, a cancer patient, and a caregiver, you get MAJOR PSYCHO!

PET scans show more than CT scans. However, thanks to insurance in most cases, CT scans have to be performed before PET due to the expense of the test.

When you read a report made by the radiologist, there is certain lingo used. ALTHOUGH, COULD BE, MAY, DIFFICULT TO EXCLUDE, POSSIBLY. These words are evasive; they don't mean 100% guaranteed.

Why? Because a scan doesn't show you that it is cancer. Some things can make it look like cancer, but sometimes it isn't. For example, inflammation can fool the eye of the reader to look like cancer. So can scar tissue.

After the doctor receives the report from the radiologist, the oncologist decides what he or she thinks about the cellular activity, whether it be a mass or a lymph node. One doctor told me one time, "If it walks like a duck and quacks like a duck, it is a duck." If a surgeon can get to the area of suspicion, a biopsy will be done. If in a difficult area to reach, the oncologists will look at the scans and blood work to determine the plan of action.

Your life still somewhat revolves around cancer years after the treatment is over. Until you are five years out free from the disease, do you not worry as much? Scans are conducted during these five years. Depression decreases due to normal daily living.

However, the anxiety is still there. The result of the scan appointment is the most relaxing day after you receive good news. After that, you begin to go back to becoming PSYCHO! Thoughts take over. "Is it back?"

Demolish arguments and every pretension that sets itself up against the knowledge of God, and we take captive every thought to make it obedient to Christ.

2 Corinthians 10:5

6.

HOLD THE ROPE

Football teams that are successful have one thing in common—they hold the rope. When they hold the rope, they know that they can trust every hand that is placed there. They know that their hands will bleed for each other. They understand that if they all hold on, they will win.

When we think of the rope, we think of hope. When someone is drowning, we throw the rope. When someone is climbing the cliff, we throw the rope. We tell them to hold on tightly.

As a team, we are all rope holders. We hang on tightly for each other, and we all have one common goal. No one on the rope lets the other teammates down.

Look at all the members of your team and know they will hold the rope for you. The team holds the rope when the going gets tough. They work on all the plays together. They won't let go.

Everyone on the rope knows their job, and they execute. Each person holds the rope for each other. Cancer, the opponent, will try to take you off the rope, but with all hands on the rope, the team becomes one force holding on for each other.

Cancer doesn't respect you; you have to make cancer earn your respect. You must outcompete cancer. With everyone holding onto the rope you can outplay cancer.

The Huddle

Huddle up! The huddle is where you build your cancer team. This is almost as important as the head coach and you as the patient. You are going to be dealing with your doctors and your caregiver every day. You are on the receiving end of your team's efforts. You have to make sure that your whole team is holding onto the same rope.

When Herm Edwards, a former player and coach, spoke to the Razorback Touchdown Club, he discussed the huddle. He said those in the huddle have the same goal. Everyone in the huddle knows their position and does their part. They are all there to go the distance for each other and are accountable to each other. In the huddle is where all the nonsense is cut out. There is one voice, and everyone listens. One person is calling the plays, and then the plays are executed. Everyone expects each other to follow the plan provided for victory. After the call is given, the huddle breaks and everyone does their job.

So what does it look like when your huddle begins to form? How do you go about putting the members of your huddle together?

Pray that God will lead you to the particular teammates that are right for you. When you begin meeting with your doctors, you will have a feeling of peace if you have the right players in place. These are five key pieces to have in your huddle:

The difference between the impossible and the possible lies in a person's determination.

Tommy Lasorda

- FOCUSED GOALS (Everyone in your huddle is focused and committed to the common purpose of winning. There isn't anyone in the huddle who isn't up to the challenge. Everyone has a winning mindset.)

- ACTIVE PARTICIPATION (Everyone works together to actively participate in your cancer plan.)

- TRUST (Everyone trusts each other and respects each other's decisions.)

- SUPPORTIVE ENVIRONMENT (Everyone encourages each other, celebrates achievements, and readjusts when necessary.)

- CLEAR COMMUNICATION (No one is intimidated by anyone within the huddle. Questions are asked and answered if possible. Input is given when needed.)

Your huddle is going to be on the field with you for every play. When they throw you the ball, you catch. They are holding the rope just as tightly as you are. Now it's time to break the huddle and play this game.

PERSONAL ESSAY

Just Do It

Don
Dad to Cancer Patient

The whole thing about cancer is interesting. You begin to read, and you read everything. There is so much to learn out there. I soon found out that when you are

82

faced with a cancer situation, people start coming to you with questions. I wasn't an expert on cancer, but because my son had cancer, I was approached by many.

I may not have had an answer to all the questions, but I had a part I played. My son is a high school basketball coach, a job I had for years. We had a unique situation because I left coaching and became principal. I am now his principal. When he was diagnosed with cancer, I didn't have time to sit back. I had to step up. That is just what I did. There wasn't anything to discuss or figure out. There wasn't a choice of yes or no. I just had to do it!

While he was out for surgery, I became the coach. Yes, I was exhausted, and I realized why I got out of coaching, but I did it for him.

There was a fine line drawn, and I had to be very cautious about me coaching his team. I wanted him to know that he was still the head coach and I was just the fill in. I wanted him to know that the decisions were still his decisions to be made. He needed to understand that things were waiting for him to get well. He had things he had to get back to doing.

Knowing this kept him grabbing at getting well. He had the choice to stand up and fight or lie down and give up. A few times he lay down, but not very often. When he was tired and exhausted, he didn't let anyone know it. Only those of us close to him knew.

He has completed all treatment and scans, and scopes are clean. Now he not only coaches his team, but he coaches others. Many people seek him out and ask him questions.

He doesn't blame anyone or anything. He doesn't sit down or lie down. He makes a choice every day to

Therefore encourage one another and build each other up, just as in fact you are doing.

1 Thessalonians
5:11

stand and fight. He makes a choice every day not just to help himself but to help others.

He makes a choice every day just to do it!

THE MVP AND THE SPECIAL TEAMS

When you break the huddle and go to work on the field, you want your oncologist to be the MVP. The MVP is the most valuable player. He/she has been awarded this prestigious honor because he/she has performed better than anyone on the field. The MVP is responsible for his/her team's success.

Don't you want an MVP who will gain success for your team? So how do we find such a player? How do we find a pro? How do we find someone who is valuable?

Many times, your general practitioner will have someone in mind. They will usually get an appointment for you. Or you may have a friend who has used an oncologist he/she would highly recommend.

When you have your first oncology appointment, it is all about communication. Before you go to that first meeting, gather all your information from previous doctors. (If you have had scopes or scans, you can get digital copies of these.) List all medications that you take and the dosage of each. It saves time if you have everything gathered. Some doctor's offices will request information before you get there so they can go ahead and look at your case. (We found it is good to have a copy.) Located in the *Scouting Report* are sheets to help you gather all of your information.

At the first meeting, have a list of questions ready for the oncologist. It is a good idea to take someone with you. It is better to have two sets of ears to hear. (Example questions are located in the *Scouting Report*.)

You want to find out how many seasons they have played and how many victories they can claim.

Don't be intimidated! Remember, this is your life. Ask any and every question. THERE ISN'T A QUESTION THAT ISN'T IMPORTANT!

No matter what, you want the most talented people, on all the special teams, working and taking care of you. You want those who have trained and continued to learn. You want those individuals who have trained under the best and learned the most. You want offense, defense, and special teams that will find a way to win the ballgame. You want the team that will score the points and make the touchdowns. You want a team that will come to life during the game and win. You want a team that will find the best play and execute them. You want a team that will complete passes and make tackles. Whether it is on the last play or the first, you want the plays that will count. When the game is on the line, you want a team that won't throw an interception. You want a team that doesn't break under pressure. You want a team that is ready for the Super Bowl and will run continuously for the win.

There may be heartbreaks or setbacks. If this happens, it is time to roll up your sleeves and get to work. It is the way you handle adversity that matters. If you fall, get up.

After you've asked the general questions and decided on your oncologist, you will be given your game plan. This game plan can include one or more of the following: surgery, chemotherapy, radiation, or immunotherapy.

The players on the field that all have the same goal. Set your goals high, and don't stop till you get there.

Bo Jackson

85

- SURGERY—The surgical removal of cancer cells or tumors in the body.

- CHEMOTHERAPY—Medication used to kill cells and stop cell growth. There are various types of chemo. It can be given orally, by an injection, or through a vein. If it is administered through the vein (IV), your doctor may decide to put in a port. This is a line that is used to manage the medication. With a port, you don't have to have an IV started with every chemo. Chemotherapy may have side effects, but some medications help with this. People react differently, so your experience will not be the same as someone else's.

- RADIATION—X-rays that are directed at the tumor. This can be in high or low doses. If you have radiation, you will be marked with a marker so that the rays will be directed toward the specific target. You may also be fitted with a shield to protect other parts of your body. There may be side effects of radiation. As our doctors have explained to us, before radiation, you are working with a full battery, but radiation zaps you and decreases your battery. You will have fatigue. Patients will react differently, depending on the dosage and where in the body the radiation is presented.

- IMMUNOTHERAPY—This is fairly new and works by using a person's immune system in fighting cancer. It can also be called biologic therapy or biotherapy. Immunotherapy either trains the immune system to attack cancer cells or it boosts the body's immune system. Immunotherapy works better on some types of cancer than others. The AMERICAN CANCER SOCIETY has information on its website (www.cancer.org) that explains all the details of immunotherapy.

Depending on the plan of action, you may end up with a surgeon and a radiologist. More than likely, you will end up with some special teams. If you have surgery, you will have your special team surgeon, and if you have radiation, you will have your special team radiologist. If you have to have surgery, your oncologist will recommend one for you, BUT you get to choose. You can always get a second opinion on anything and everything. It is your choice what doctor treats your body. You need to have complete confidence in your team of physicians.

My son-in-law had to decide what surgeon he was going to use. He met with one who was a general surgeon. They asked many questions. After the question/answer session, the doctor looked at them and said, "Feel free to get a second opinion." He even gave them a doctor's name. They then met with the second physician. They chose the first doctor, who, as it turns out had conferred with the second doctor to make sure he was making the correct decisions. That is the kind of doctor you want—the one who says to you, "get a second opinion," then checks with the other doctors to make sure he is doing the correct protocol.

OTHER SPECIAL TEAMS

Besides your surgeon special team and your radiologist special team, you may decide to have other special teams to help you along the way. These people are part

Two are better than one, because they have a good return for their labor: If either of them falls down, one can help the other up. But pity anyone who falls and has no one to help them up. Also, if two lie down together, they will keep warm. But how can one keep warm alone? Though one may be overpowered, two can defend themselves. A cord of three strands is not quickly broken.

Ecclesiastes 4:9-12

of the alternative treatment special teams. These treatment options are listed under Naturopathic Medicine. Naturopathic Medicine is used to treat a patient as a whole in a non-toxic way. It is the use of therapeutic methods and substances that promote self-healing.

Before going into the details of alternative medicine, let me say that I am in no way a medical professional, and this does not mean you should not do traditional treatment. My intent is not to diagnose, prescribe, or make any medical claims. However, there are choices available to help with healing. Many of these treatments contribute to calm the mind, body, and soul allowing your body to take full advantage of the medical treatment being used to treat your disease.

Many cancer centers offer a variety of these alternative therapies. The cancer centers' social workers will be able to tell you what is available. Massage therapists, counselors, and physical therapists are some that are usually located in a cancer center.

Naturopathic medicine includes:
- Herbal and botanical preparations
- Dietary supplements
- Homeopathic remedies
- Physical therapy and exercise therapy
- Hydrotherapy
- Lifestyle counseling
- Acupuncture
- Chiropractic care

ESSENTIAL OILS

Essential oils began in biblical times. God created healing substances. These substances were found within plants. They are called essential because they are the life blood of the plant. Without these oils, the plant wouldn't have life.

In Philippians 4:18, St. Paul refers to "a fragrant offering" as an acceptable gift "and pleasing to God," which is a reference to the aromas of the essential oils used in incense, anointing oils, and sacrifices of worship. Because essential oils were created by God, they do not have side effects like our medications of today. They are non-toxic, harmless to human tissue, and promote healing. There are six ways that essentials oils support us:

- As fighters against unfriendly microbes
- As balancers of bodily functions
- As raisers of our bodily frequencies
- As antioxidants that purify our systems
- As clearers of negative emotional baggage
- As uplifters of our spiritual awareness

In today's world, several companies extract oil directly from the plant. These oils are recognized as the most effective medicine known to mankind. As David Stewart puts it in his book, *Oils of the Bible*, "The sun is the sole source of sunshine whether we believe in it or not. God is the sole source of healing whether we realize it or not."

There are three different ways to use these oils. It is crucial to interpret the therapeutic effects and develop a personal holistic health regime. The three ways are topical, aromatic, and internal.

When applying an oil topically, you should use one to three drops, usually diluted with a carrier oil such as fractionated coconut oil. The oil is massaged into parts of the body that have the largest pores. The

Is anyone among you sick? Let them call the elders of the church to pray over them and anoint them with oil in the name of the Lord.

James 5:14

feet are the second fastest area of the body to absorb oils, also behind the ears and on the wrists.

Aromatically essential oils can do what many medications cannot. The easiest and simplest way is to use them is with a diffuser that spreads a mist in the air. You can also have direct inhalation. When essential oils are breathed, the aroma can travel through the back of the nasal passage and penetrate the blood brain barrier. The part of the brain that doesn't understand words can respond to the smell and fragrance of the essential oil. Penetrating the blood brain barrier is something that medications cannot do.

Only pure therapeutic-grade essential oils should be used for internal consumption. The FDA has given some essential oils approval. When consuming essential oils, they should either be used sublingually, placed in a capsule, added to a beverage, or used while cooking. Essential oils are stronger than the herb or the spice because they come directly from the plant, so a little goes a long way.

PERSONAL ESSAY

LOOK INTO IT—YOU NEVER KNOW
Cheerleader

Right after my brother-in-law was diagnosed with brain cancer, I went to an essential oils class. The instructor gave a summary of the book *Healing Oils of the Bible*. After that, she explained Doterra oils. These oils come directly from the plant in its origin. For example, rosemary is native to the Mediterranean region; therefore, rosemary oil is extracted from the rosemary plant in that area.

90

I was amazed at all the information about the essential oils. When I thought about Biblical times and how they didn't have a pharmacy to get medicines, it made perfect sense. People were healed in the Bible—some by miracles, but some were healed by using biblical medicines, which were essential oils.

After the workshop, I called my sister-in-law. I knew she was going to be skeptical. She was in the medical field, actually a pharmaceutical rep, so I knew it was going to take some convincing. I shared with her everything I learned and just said, "Why don't you look into it?"

She started reading and researching. She attended essential oil meetings. After learning all the details, she began using a Doterra blend called DDR PRIME. DDR PRIME is an oil for healthy cellular integrity. It is a combination of oils that provide powerful antioxidants. It contains clove, thyme, and wild orange. It also includes oils from frankincense, lemongrass, summer savory, and niaouli. You can use it in different ways. My sister-in-law began taking a capsule, breaking it, and rubbing the oil on her husband's feet. She has been doing this for three years.

Glioblastoma is a terminal illness. My brother-in-law's was stage 3 at diagnosis. Yes, he did the medical cancer regimen, but he also added essential oils. He is still alive today three years later. He is a miracle maybe not because of the oils, but you never know.

Success is determined by everyone working together strategically to give your team the best chance to win.

Misti Coker

91

MOMENTS

Amy
Daughter of Cancer Patient, APN for Many

I am a medical professional, and it is from that perspective that I hope to give you an idea of how I view life, illness, and death.

I was 13 and at cheer camp when on a pay phone I heard my mom say the word "malignant." I suppose that word wasn't as explicit as "cancer." THAT word I would have understood. We did not have cell phones, computers, or Google to help me better understand the definition. Terminal, end stage, or even hopeless would have been a better way to describe it to a teenager.

Five months later, my daddy died in our home from lung cancer. The priest came to our home, the family arrived at our home, and long after he was gone, an ambulance arrived at our home. You see, he had to be pronounced "dead" and have a death certificate signed by a doctor or coroner. When EMS arrived, they found him pulseless and cold; they began CPR and full resuscitative efforts. I remember them saying this was their "protocol" as my mother and uncle screamed at them that he was gone. A peaceful death had turned into a chaotic, confusing end to cancer. I remember thinking, "Where was this urgent medical care and intervention when he was fighting cancer?" Funny how death will get undivided attention and LIFE doesn't.

This was when I decided I wanted to help people when they felt most helpless. You can impact a person's life even when the message is not the one you want to give.

We all have those moments in life that we will never forget. Usually the place, the day, the hour, and the season when our life changed is engraved into our memory. So, I thought, why can't God send someone to us to make "that moment" more bearable, or at least leave a loving memory to accompany the tragedy? As we all know, this is not always the case. We usually feel as if we are drowning without anyone to save us. We hang on to every word hoping it will be something profound to make our hurt tolerable.

So, I want to tell you about healthcare providers. All kinds—MD's, NP's, RN's, surgeons, oncologists, therapists, etc., etc., etc.

We are all HUMANS! Some brilliant beyond imagination, but still HUMAN! Capable of having a bad day, capable of making mistakes, capable of saying the wrong thing HUMAN. Which is why I am telling you that your hope for the best care is that your healthcare providers are humble, empathetic, kind, and have faith in GOD.

If I told you I am afraid when I care for your child, would you bring them to me as a patient? Probably not—but you should. You should be thankful that my biggest fear is that I will have a bad day and miss the smallest detail that could mean the difference in your child's health.

I remember a radiologist more than 20 years ago telling me about a profound moment in his career. He was reading a mammogram of a woman who would later be told she had breast cancer. The tumor was visible on the film to the naked eye. Then he showed me the films from the previous mammogram. I didn't see a thing. He then showed me a tiny dot, close to

Though he may stumble, he will not fall, for the Lord upholds him with his hand.

Psalm 37:24

the size of a ballpoint pen dot. He said, "it was there, and I missed it." HUMAN. He went on to tell me of how he sobbed when he discovered it. He carried those films with him in his briefcase to remind him of the lives that he impacted each day. He has since lost his life to cancer, but his lesson lives on. On my hectic days, I have to remind myself that I might be one of those engraved memories to someone, and I would rather be afraid than arrogant.

So, on any given day, I will choose to be of average intelligence—but prayerfully empathetic, attentive, and patient.

I have seen miracles many times in my career. Many before I even understood what I was experiencing in a young life. I worked at Arkansas Children's Hospital (ACH) in the Neonatal Intensive Care Unit (NICU) long before I became a parent. Bedside vigils of parents were commonplace, and I remember wondering how they went without sleep and why they would never leave. Even though their infant had the best doctors and nurses caring for them, their resilience was out of fear that if they left for one moment, something would change. Of course, after I became a mother, what was initially sympathy became empathy and it all made perfect sense.

I am brought to my knees when I think of a patient, whom I prayed for God to take and to give peace to the family. His mom was a teacher and his dad an adult Intensive Care Unit nurse, and their prayers far surpassed my brief ones. You see, this was their one and only child. He was born weighing more than nine pounds—perfect—but quickly developed persistent fetal circulation (PFC) and was transported by helicop-

94

ter to ACH. Over the course of many months, I cannot count the number of times he coded (died) and was brought back to life. His parents and grandparents said their final goodbyes one evening behind screens hours before my last shift. Prayers continued for a miracle despite a hopeless situation. The next morning, you can imagine my surprise when he was still alive. There was no logical, medical, or understandable explanation. We had NICU reunions, and years later, the infant that I prayed to go to heaven played baseball, got straight As, and was a beautiful blond-headed, blue-eyed boy. Thank God for my unanswered prayer.

I went on to be a flight nurse and, as you can imagine, experienced more adrenaline, exhaustion, and miracles than ever before. Heartbreak was very present—but so were hope and happiness, as well.

The image of an unconscious boy with meningitis, pale in color and seemingly lifeless late one night, was transformed into a voice and a pitter patter of feet running down the hall of the hospital yelling "Captain, my captain and angel." I cannot rationalize how he survived or how he had any memory of me when he was unconscious the entire flight.

The next morning when I watched the sunrise above the clouds in flight, I knew it was the closest to heaven or being an angel that I would ever experience in this life. I can't help but wonder, while we are trying to get closer to heaven, if we should pay more attention to the fact that God may be reaching down to meet us half way.

More than 12 years after hundreds of flights, I had a "moment." I was seeing an infant in what is now my slower paced clinic day. The grandmother said, "You

Do right. Do your best. Treat others, as you want to be treated.

Lou Holtz

probably don't remember us—but we will never forget you. You transported my grandson after he was born."

She then showed me a picture of a red-headed, freckle-faced boy grinning ear to ear. This is one of those moments when your heart falls. Did I say the right thing? Did I give them the hope they needed? And most of all, was God with me?

Anyone with healthcare experiences can tell you the good, the bad, and the ugly. But it is my hope that I and ALL those who provide health care will remember that this could be "a moment" in time. I always want to be "afraid"—I always want to be "sad" or "happy" with the news I have to share with you. If my emotions leave me, then so has my compassion. If I do not understand that God is the ultimate healer and I am not, then take me out of my profession. If I do not count prayer, faith, and hope as part of my prescriptions and advice, then take away the medicine and tests as well. If healing does not include your spirit, your heart, and your body, then your strength will not likely be present. I believe all these things to be instrumental in healing.

The Quarterback

Your quarterback may not be the most knowledgeable on the field; however, he or she knows what plays need to be in your best interest. He has your playbook memorized. He processes all of your information and synthesizes it so you will receive the best care and the outcome will be successful. He has the ability to make decisions for you and with you. He tends to be emotionally strong and is a valuable asset to your team.

He is your armor and always has your back. He never lets anyone or anything hurt you. He knows what works best for you. He carries you off the playing field when you need to be carried.

Your quarterback isn't on the sidelines; he is right beside you on the field. He is happy when you are happy and sad when you are sad. If you fall back, he is always there to catch you. As stated earlier, he has your back and you have his.

If you haven't figured it out, the quarterback is your caregiver, and you can't play this game without him (or her).

If you are a caregiver reading this, I hope this helps you and gives you information that will help you on the playing field.

You can and will be a game changer. It is very time consuming, trying, and emotional. Just as the patient is going through changes, you as the caregiver are going through changes as well. There are new worries and added responsibilities. Not only are you trying to take on the new role of being a caregiver for your loved one, you are also doing what you have always done. Your income may change and your dreams for the future may shift as well. You have to realize that you cannot do it all, and at times, even the caregiver needs a caregiver.

As I talked to caregivers, one young lady's comments stand out in my mind. She said, "When my mother received the news that she had cancer, I was shocked, but after looking back, cancer allowed me to spend more quality time with my mother. If it hadn't been for her cancer, I would have not made time every day to be with her."

THE CAREGIVER IS THE SILENT SUFFERER, REMAINING SILENT WHEN THEY NEED TO SCREAM.

Watching my daughter, I realized that the care-giver goes through stages, much like the stages of grief. I want to emphasize that these feelings are normal. The realization that you are going through these stages is the first step to being able to walk through them. There is no time limit and no particular order that these feelings will occur. You may not go through them exactly like another caregiver. These feelings can also come and go and shift back and forth. I also found that my son-in-law went through similar emo-tions as the patient.

When her husband was first diagnosed, my daugh-ter was in shock. This protected her from emotional trauma. How could this be happening? The next phase was that of denial. This can't be true. As they got into their cancer routine, my daughter didn't have to care for her husband 24 hours a day. After the crisis phase had passed and my daughter had time to think, she became angry. She was angry because her life had changed and she had to find a new normal at such a young age. She became angry at herself and even her spouse. The next stage is depression when guilt sets in and the past feelings you have had make you upset. You may even think you should have done something to prevent the cancer. Then come the tears as sadness sets in, and there are feelings of loneliness and emptiness. You want your old life back, the life before cancer. After these stages comes the acceptance, the acceptance of the cancer and the question of what God's plan will be.

There are also physical symptoms that come with caring for someone, such as increased fatigue, headaches, insomnia, and other aches and pains. After all of this, you will find a renewed hope. After the treatments, surgery, and any other medical procedures, the weight will be lifted, and you can see a hope for the future.

Remember this: EVEN THE CAREGIVER NEEDS A CAREGIVER. To be a good caregiver, you have to understand how your body is feeling. You must take care of your physical and mental needs. Write a journal, visit a therapist, or find a support group. You may even need to get on anxiety or depression medication, and there is nothing wrong with that. Begin by making a list of people who can help you, such as neighbors, church members, co-workers, family members, and friends. This will become your team. People want to help, but many are waiting for you to reach out to them. YOU NEED A TEAM TO GATHER A TEAM FOR YOU!

Time Out

During every game of life every player needs a time out. No matter what role you are playing, you need time set aside for a break.

When we are facing adversity, emotions can be overwhelming and can flood the body, especially our brains. When this happens, our bodies will react to the stressor. Because of the extra anxiety, your body needs time to be calm. This calming of your body and brain can make a difference in the outcome.

It will bring you benefits when you set aside time for the time out. The noisiness of the game can cause us to worry and stress, but time outs can bring a positive impact on your ability to cope. Disconnecting for a short time can rejuvenate and refresh your body.

You may be saying there is no way you can do this. I am here to tell you, "YOU HAVE TO TAKE A

When people don't take time out, they stop being productive.

Carisa Bianchi

THE
CAREGIVER
EXECUTES ALL
THE PLAYS
GIVEN TO THEM
AND CARRIES
ALL THE
BURDENS. IT'S
OKAY TO TAKE
A TIME OUT.

TIME OUT." You don't have to go anywhere; you can find a quiet place in your home or in your yard. You may have to just get in your car and drive around. You need it and deserve it! You need your own personal pep rally to get pumped back up for the rest of the game.

When you don't take a time out, you can cause more harm on your body, even if you are healthy. Time outs prevent stress-induced illnesses. Stress can do harm to our bodies, sometimes even more damage than cancer.

Everyone is different, so your personal pep rally won't look like someone else's. Here are some things to think about:

- Where is your favorite place?
- What is your favorite thing to do?
- What is your favorite restaurant?
- What would take all the noisiness out of your world and bring quiet?

Set a new goal to have a time out. You aren't halting; you are just taking a breather. Find this time to encourage gratitude, cultivate joy, breathe, smile, and be happy. Time outs give you the motivation you need to get back in the game and move down the field.

PERSONAL ESSAY

MILES WITH THE MONSTER

Teddy
Caregiver, husband

Early in November 2011, Barbara was traveling 60 miles from our home to her destination. She was then to go south 70 miles. However, she ended up going north. She called me to give her directions. Barbara ended up stopping at a mall to shop. When she was ready to depart, she wasn't sure which way to go. She called me again, and I gave her directions. An hour later she called again, and she had missed a turn. Once again, I gave her directions. I waited on her at a local restaurant, but she never got there.

When I called again, she was back 10 miles from her first location. I told her, "I'm coming to get you!" Barbara responded, "No I can get home!" A little while later I called, and she was headed north on another interstate that would eventually have taken her out of Arkansas.

It was at this point that I decided I was going to find my wife. I prayed that there would be a state trooper somewhere on the highway. When I pulled up to a small rural town, a police officer pulled up next to me. My prayer had been answered. I informed the officer, and the officer put out an alert. They found Barbara at the exit where I had told her to stop. The officer stayed with her until I was able to get there.

Seven hours and more than 200 miles Barbara had driven. The monster that was now traveling with her no matter where she went confused her. There were many miles ahead for Barbara and me. Many miles that only God could get us through.

As I sat and listened to Teddy, I saw the passion he had for taking care of his wife. The struggle was there, and the heaviness still lingered even though she was gone. He discussed every date and every detail of Barbara's cancer. He shared with me how God spoke to him over and over. At times he would listen, but

To the world you may be one person, but to one person you may be the world.

Dr. Seuss

101

sometimes he would take the advice of those in the bleachers. Teddy learned quickly that as the caregiver you know best. You are there in the huddle with the patient at all times. You know what they need. You can tell by their voice and their physical appearance how they are. You know when they need visitors and when they don't. As the caregiver, you are the manager of everything, and everyone else should follow your lead.

Teddy decided early on that his house was going to be full of faith. Only those who were faith driven were allowed on this journey with him and Barbara. For miraculous healing, everyone had to be of one accord. So as the caregiver, you must deal with all of the defensive players coming at you. It can be difficult, but only positive attitudes can drive you through cancer.

God led Teddy. There were several situations that Teddy inquired that God spoke directly to him. One was in the very beginning. Insurance refused to pay for a scan. God woke Teddy in the middle of the night and told him to look at the policy. He looked and saw that if Barbara were to go to the ER, she could receive a scan. The next day Teddy went head to head with personnel. They finally said, "Sir, take her to the ER." To the ER they went, and the scan was completed. At another time during her illness, Barbara became very depressed. She didn't want to get out of bed nor did she want to walk anywhere. God told Teddy to put up pictures of their family, everyone. Teddy listened and filled their home with pictures. Barbara went from barely moving to sprinting.

God had given Teddy an assignment. That assignment was to take care of Barbara. That is what he did.

He knew that God was with him. God never left him. He was with him for every mile of the journey.

Teddy knew when Barbara took her last breath that she had finished her assignment on Earth. He knew he had to continue miles without her, but her legacy lives on through him and the many people she touched during her miles on this earth.

That monster may have taken Barbara, but he couldn't take the miles of goodness she left behind.

Doctors diagnose, nurses heal, and caregivers make sense out of it all.

Brett H. Lewis

THE KICKERS

The kickers on a team may be treated as an afterthought. They aren't in the game as much as the other positions. They are in the backfield not speaking up when things go wrong or when things go badly; however, when something is their fault, they hear about it. Kickers have to learn how to adapt. They must kick the ball through a small opening, and at times it can be a long distance.

Fans think that being the kicker is an easy job. The ball is placed, the kicker runs up to it, and then he strikes it with a foot. There are no plays to remember, just kick. However, there are more things that go into kicking beside just kicking the ball. There are techniques that a kicker must perfect, and they must have a narrow focus at all times. One major factor that affects a kick is the weather. Hopefully, the wind is blowing with the kick, but sometimes you have to kick against the wind. Weather conditions affect the kicker's approach and stability and how the ball flies through the air.

Children of cancer patients become like the kickers on the field of play. They aren't in on all the plays, so at times they don't know all of the details. They are left in the backfield. What used to seem to be a normal childhood life has quickly shifted to the abnormal. They are now dealing with a crosswind that is wreaking havoc. Children must learn how to relate and adjust to the new resistance in their life. They now have to live within the boundaries that cancer has made for them. They must go against the wind until it decides to subside.

In an article written by Laura Nathan-Garner, "When a Parent Has Cancer: Helping Teens and Kids Cope," she recommends the five C's when discussing the dreaded C word.

- Say that it's Cancer.
- Tell your kids, "You didn't Cause it. You can't Catch it. You can't Control it."
- Tell your kids that you Can still spend quality time together, participate in care, still be a kid, have fun, etc.

Here are some other things she suggested:

- Stick to a routine.
- Be honest.
- Find someone to help.
- Try to maintain regular parent/child roles and responsibilities as much as possible.
- Let your children express themselves, maybe through a journal.

Cancer.org has an e-book that is awesome: *Helping Children When a Family Member Has Cancer*. This e-book explains many areas that children need to know. It discusses how to handle when a parent has cancer and what to do when it may not be a parent. For instance, it may be a sibling who has cancer.

Cancercare.org suggests:

- Prepare what you are going to say.
- Set the tone. How you say it can be as important as what you say.
- Consider the age of your child.
- Explain treatment plans and how it will affect their lives.
- Answer your child's questions as accurately as possible.
- Reassure your children they can't catch cancer.
- Let them know they have a support system and who their support system is.
- Allow your children to participate in your care.
- Encourage your children to express their feelings.
- Reassure your children that they will be cared for.
- Make communicating a priority.
- Show your child lots of love and affection.
- Ask a professional for help.

The first conversation about cancer is the most difficult. You as the parent know your child better than anyone. You will know what works for your child. Follow your instinct on how to handle everything. Don't feel bad saying no to what others think your child needs. Even though you have cancer, you still know best.

Not looking to your own interests but each of you to the interests of the others.

Philippians 2:4

AGE IS EVERYTHING

Mom
Cancer Patient

My daughter knows nothing else but me being sick. I have had cancer her whole life. When visiting about how to handle what you tell a child when a parent has cancer, these were my thoughts:

- Age is everything. What you say depends on the age of the child. When my daughter was four, we would say momma is sick. The older she has gotten, the more details we have told her, mainly because we don't want her to hear from someone else. Also, the older she has gotten, she will ask more questions. At first, we didn't say cancer, but now we do.

- My daughter began asking about my cancer when her school started praying for people with cancer. It was then when she would ask, "Is cancer bad? Can someone die of cancer?" We explain how everyone's cancer is different. We don't include all the nitty gritty. We are honest, we say what we feel she needs to hear, and we answer her questions to the best of our ability.

- The people who have helped me the most with this subject are the social workers. They gave me a lot of information on how to talk to your child when you have cancer. Social workers are resourceful. They have material that your child can color and learn from.

- When our daughter was younger, we would take her with us since I have to go out of state for surgery. Our parents would go to help. We didn't like leaving her for weeks at a time, and we realized that if we were gone for long periods, her personality would change somewhat. She would have some anger and meltdowns. Change in behavior is normal with any child when their routine has been altered. Staying at grandparent's homes instead of being at home with mom and dad on their regular schedule can affect a child. As she has gotten older, she doesn't want to miss school. We don't take her with us as often. Sometimes our parents will bring her to visit on the weekends. Once again this is determined by age.

You are the parent. You know your child better than anyone else. Use your best judgment and let your actions be determined by the age of your child or children. In spite of cancer, try to take time to get away from cancer. Try to chisel in family fun time. By doing this, your child will recognize how much you care about them.

Do not be anxious about anything, but in every situation, by prayer and petition, with thanksgiving, present your requests to God. And the peace of God, which transcends all understanding, will guard your hearts and your minds in Christ Jesus.

Philippians 4:6-7

PERSONAL ESSAY

THE SHIFT

Lana
Sister of Cancer Patient

When I was 15 and my brother was seven, he was diagnosed with leukemia. That was when my life changed. I had to become an adult quickly. It was natural to me. Since my mom was gone with my brother at times, I just had to take over. My grandparents would stay with me when my mom and dad were both gone. When my dad would come home, he would tell me, "Your mom needs these things when I go back." It was easy for me to gather just what she needed.

I went to school 20 miles away from home, and I didn't drive yet, so I had to make arrangements to get to school and get home. I learned how to plan and how to be organized. I had to have a plan on how I was getting to this activity and that activity. Sometimes I would even ask my friends if their parents could take me to the store. When I would ask this, I would get strange looks from my friends. At 15, no one else was having to do the grocery shopping.

My job had shifted from high school student to a job I never thought I would have at 15. I didn't mind, and my parents knew they didn't have to worry about me. I filled in for my mom. I paid the bills and took care of anything she needed.

Today, at 32 and 24, I still tease my brother and tell him he is the favorite. My mom says he isn't the favorite. She just knows I can take care of myself.

I am the way I am because of the shift. I am independent. I plan ahead. I am in charge of many things. Almost every club that I am a member I am president. I know that I get things done, and other people know that about me.

Others probably don't know the real reason why I am wired the way I am, but it is something I will never forget.

The shift is what made me the person I am today.

THE CHEERLEADER

A cheerleader is a dreamer who never gives up.

The cheerleader isn't in the huddle or on the field, but he/she is part of the team. He/she is on the sidelines ready and waiting to call a cheer. The cheerleader may be the parent of the caregiver or a very close friend or relative. The cheerleader's main responsibility is to be ready at any time to motivate. He/she is there to help you laugh or to be a shoulder to cry on. The cheerleader knows what you need and when you need it. They are ready to perform tasks— no matter what it is or how much time it takes. They will go the extra mile to keep everyone comfortable.

Cheerleaders usually wait on their captain to call the play, so if you are the patient or the caregiver, give your cheerleader direction. They are there for you, so tell them what to do. Let them know exactly what you need.

I know exactly the role of the cheerleader. I am my daughter's cheerleader. I wanted to fix the situation, just like mothers do, but there was no easy fix. All I could do was be there for my daughter. I began to realize what type of day she was going to have by how her husband was feeling. If he was anxious, she was anxious. If she was tired, it was worse. She was still working, getting her master's degree, doing household duties, and helping him. She was on overload. I didn't wait to be told what to do, and usually when you have a close relationship with the caregiver, you don't have to wait. Just jump right in. I have listed things that I did to keep my daughter motivated and to try to keep the stress level low.

This is what I found to work well. These small acts of kindness helped out tremendously:

- Sent texts just saying, "What can I do for you?"
- Cleaned the house
- Went to the grocery store
- Made meals to be placed in the freezer
- Washed laundry
- Went through bills and paid them
- Called insurance companies
- Gave her a day off
- Took her to dinner
- Took her shopping
- Took her to the Sonic Drive-in for a drink, drove around, and listened to her
- Set up a motivation mailing list with her friends and my friends. Everyone had his or her day to mail something. It went through the whole 10 weeks of treatment.
- Sometimes something simple and easy is best.

PERSONAL ESSAY

Fix It

Misti Cheerleader
Story located within the pages of 1 Heart Mom, Relevant Pages Press

Her crystal blue eyes looked at me as if she were three years old again. The expression she carried was saying, "Momma, fix it!"

The doctor had just rounded the corner and told us the news. The information that we didn't want to hear, nor that the doctor thought he was going to find.

Cancer! That small, six-letter word that changes lives forever. Cancer is an atrocious word for anyone's ears, but to young newlyweds, it is unthinkable.

My daughter's husband had begun having trouble swallowing. It had gone on for months. She told him to go to the doctor, but he put it off. It gradually got worse. One thing led to another. Food wouldn't go down, and he felt that liquid was just dripping. He lost 15 pounds in a week. We knew something was wrong; however, we thought maybe just a procedure to stretch the esophagus would work. Through the help of others, they got an appointment with a gastroenterologist who immediately scheduled an esophagogastroduodenoscope (EGD).

I didn't have to go, but as a mother, I didn't want my daughter to sit alone as her husband had this procedure. After the procedure had been finished, we all waited anxiously for the outcome. We asked if he could swallow better. We wanted him to say, "Of course, I can," but he answered, "I'm not sure."

When the doctor rounded the corner, I knew by the look on his face it wasn't good. As he began speaking, I realized we were wrong. It wasn't going to be a quick and easy fix. When the doctor said he had found a mass, my daughter began to ask questions, and my mind shifted into "fix-it-Momma mode." What can I do? What can I say? How can I make this better? How can I fix it?

On that hot first day of July, my daughter and her husband were thrown into a storm, and they couldn't simply click their ruby red slippers three times and get out of Kansas. They were in the eye of the hurricane, and the winds and water were swirling around them. They were drowning, or at least they thought they were. They were sinking, sinking deeper in the troubled waters. From one doctor's appointment to another, the information got scarier. My daughter, being a nurse, knew and understood everything that the doctors were saying, and that scared her even more. So many rounds of chemo, so many treatments of radiation, and then a surgery that is profound. Removal of a rib and puncturing of a lung was followed by a long hospital stay. The road was long, and the journey was going to be a tough one.

Questions began filling my daughter's brain. Was he going to survive? Were the treatments going to make him more ill? How was she going to continue working a 12-hour afternoon-to-morning shift at the children's hospital? How was she going to continue her schoolwork in nurse practitioner's school? How were they going to pay the bills? Were they going to be able to have children after all the treatments? How did this happen? What is God trying to tell me? What am I going to do? Why? What? When? How?

As my daughter looked for answers, she would turn to me expecting me to have some brilliant explanation. I, too, like her was not only scared but horrified! However, being the mother and cheerleader, I couldn't let her know my fears. All I could do was be her life preserver. She had fallen off the boat into the deep dark waters, and I needed to wrap my arms around her and save her.

As I write this, raindrop tears are dripping down my checks. My emotions are raw, and my body is weak from worry. I question, just as my daughter questions. God, why can't I fix this, or why won't you help me fix it? I know that is a rhetorical question, but I still want to ask. I want to be more than a life preserver. I want to be the miracle worker. I want to say a few words, and it all be gone for good with no recurrence.

No matter how old our children are, when they fall and scrape their knees, we are there, and it is our natural instinct to go straight into fix-it mode. When we become mothers, we can never reverse the role and become non-mothers. Once we have given birth and our title becomes a mom, our job starts and never ends. It isn't like we can hit the time clock and clock out.

The clock was still ticking, and I still wanted to fix the storm. I yearned for the day when my daughter was little, and she had small worries. I wanted to pick her up, hold her tight, and say, "I will fix it." But that wasn't going to happen. I wish for her life to be pain-free. I want her and her husband to celebrate and do what young married couples do. I want her to start planning for a family. BUT, and that is a word I like and dislike, cancer has invited itself in and plans to stay a while, and the only thing I can do is be committed to my daughter.

We, as mothers, are dedicated to our children. We have a level of commitment that is beyond what anyone who isn't a mother can comprehend. It all begins the moment they begin to form within us. We carry our children for nine months, protecting them within our wombs, feeding them with nutrients so they will be ready to take that first breath when they enter the world. It doesn't stop after birth. We help them crawl, walk, and then run. We teach them about the world. We share our experiences, hoping they will learn from us. We support them, build self-esteem, and love them unconditionally. We let them fall to be able to teach them how to get back up.

A MEMBER OF

THE TEAM,

SUPPORTER,

ENTHUSIASTIC

AND VOCAL,

TOUGH,

HARDWORKING,

YOUR FOCUS IS

ON THE TEAM.

Our job is non-stop, 24 hours a day. Our job is during the light of day and during the dark of night. Our job just isn't during the good times, but also the bad. We are there during the happy and glorious times, but also during the pain and the sorrow. Any emotion that has surfaced or is hidden from the world, we are aware of it. This job of motherhood can bring joy and heartache. It can be overwhelming, but it is a gift. It may not always be wrapped up with the perfect bow; however, it is what makes life colorful. Mothers aren't paid in cash; we are paid in love.

My momma job now included cancer—something I had prayed wouldn't bless us with its presence. So, what was my new job description going to consist of? I started asking questions again.

Since I couldn't fix it, what could I do as a mother? What could I do to ease the pain? What could I do to relieve some worry?

It was time for me to suit up and go out on the field of play. Just like a football game against your toughest opponent, this job was going to be a tough one. This cancer game was going to be filled with first downs and setbacks, along with touchdowns and fumbles. I had to put on all my armor and come up with some trick plays. I had on my cheerleading uniform, and I was gripping my pompoms.

With that being said, I began every day with prayer. I would find myself not only praying first thing in the morning but every time I thought of my daughter and her husband. "Pray without ceasing" was my new motto against the enemy. I also set my personal goal for them. My goal was to bring joy to every day whether it was through something large or something

114

small. I had set a goal, and I was pushing toward the goal line. I began by gathering my team and getting them all to huddle up. I recruited my friends, her friends, and our family, and we became the EMTs (EMERGENCY MOTIVATIONAL TEAM) for my daughter and her husband. I assigned everyone a date wherein they would send any little surprise. My daughter still doesn't know I did it, but MOMS have lots of trick plays up their sleeves. I created a motivational wall out of metal in their kitchen where they could put stickers and cards. They could hang uplifting items with magnets. I cleaned, I went to the grocery store, I cooked, and I made motivational, positive posters. I took them to dinner, gave them spending change, and sent them flowers and cards, but the most important thing I did was to become a large listening ear.

I have to be honest. Many days and nights I cry. I cry because I can't fix it. I cry because I'm sad. I cry because I'm fearful that cancer may creep back in. I'm terrified that I can't prevent the things to come, heartbreak and pain. I have to be strong even though I am weak. I have to smile even though behind my smile are tears. I yearn for my daughter not to have to deal with cancer. BUT I can't fix it; all I can do is be the life preserver. All I can do is let her know, without a doubt, that she can count on me. I am here 24/7!

THE FAN

As I watched the intense basketball game between two rivals, I noticed the fans. There were those who had on the fan gear from head to toe, those who wore the colors, and then there were the fans who just

CHEERLEADERS MAY NOT LOOK LIKE A CHEERLEADER. NEVER UNDERESTIMATE THE ABILITY OF A CHEERLEADER.

A GOOD

CHEERLEADER

IS NOT

MEASURED BY

THE HEIGHT OF

HER JUMPS BUT

BY THE SPAN

OF HER SPIRIT.

came to socialize. Some fans were on fire for the team, standing and yelling during the whole game. Some who were lukewarm were standing and sitting in spurts. Then there were the cold ones—not interested. I wondered, "Why are they even here?"

A cancer patient has similar fans. There are some who are on fire for you; they jump in and get busy without being asked. Then there are the timid ones who really don't know what to do, or they are unsure what to say, so they are standoffish until someone asks them to help. Then you have the fans who are just nosey. They only cheer you on when you post something on social media.

No matter what fans you have, don't worry; there is room for all of them in the bleachers.

I have learned that most fans are in the middle category. They are in an awkward position. They want to help their team, but to be honest, they don't know what to do. They are scared they will say or do the wrong thing. At times, they can be standoffish and reluctant to jump in.

My daughter said, "If fans just do what they do best, that can really help. If their expertise is in the insurance field, help with insurance. If they cook, cook. If they are good with words, share words."

This is exactly what two of our family friends did. When my daughter's husband was diagnosed, one of her friends spent two hours explaining insurance. When my sister-in-law's husband was diagnosed, her friend took over all the bill paying.

We have made it simple for you if you are the patient or if you are a fan. In the *Scouting Report*, there is a sheet for you to fill out to give to a fan. Do not feel bad telling the fan what you need or want. This is what most fans have a difficult time with. They want to help, but they need to be directed on how to help. If you are a fan and you are reading this, we are going to give you pointers on what you can do.

- Organize a fan club—a group of people willing to help when you give them something to do. Make a list of their names, numbers, and emails.
- Set up a meal train—(www.mealtrain.com) so easy to set up, all done by email
- Give gift cards—grocery store cards, gas cards, fast food (any card is good).
- Set up your own fundraising campaign at www.gofundme.com. People can donate anonymously. Gofundme does take a percentage, but it's easy to set up.
- You can also set up a free fundraising website at www.youcaring.com/free-fundraising.
- Fundraiser-auction-raffle. This can be done in your hometown—can be done by individuals or businesses or churches
- Motivational ideas. Find out how many weeks the patient will have treatment, then assign someone to do something motivational every week. Can just be cards.
- Volunteer to drive the patient to treatment.
- Just show up to their mow yard or rake leaves.
- Wash their car.
- Give cash.
- Pick up prescriptions.
- Sit with the patient so the caregiver can have some time away, even if for only 30 minutes.

When Moses' hands grew tired, they took a stone and put it under him and he sat on it. Aaron and Hur held his hands up—one on one side, one on the other—so that his hands remained steady till sunset

Exodus 17:12

- Take their kids on a play date or a meal date.
- Make a meal.
- Organize a phone chain to check on the patient and caregiver.
- Give simple things like note cards, balloons, cross-word puzzles, jigsaw puzzles, coloring books, and coloring pencils
- Find out what their favorite food is at the time and make it for them.
- Give them a gift basket with goodies. (If doing chemo, lemondrops or jolly ranchers are good.)
- During the Christmas season, put up their tree or other decorations for them.
- Create a facebook page. This will keep everyone in the know and let others know what you need.
- Find out what time of day the patient needs a pick-me-up and drop by then.
- Don't talk about you. Let them talk about them and listen.
- Just be a listening ear.
- Follow the patient's lead.
- Do what you do best.

Be sure you check with the caregiver when giving food, flowers, or candles. Smells sometimes can be tricky, and some foods just don't taste good at the given time.

ACCESSORY AND EMBELLISHMENT

Kim
Friend

One of my dearest friends and neighbors was diagnosed with terminal brain cancer three years ago. It has robbed her and her family of many things. One of the most significant is her short-term memory.

When I first learned of the diagnosis, I was heartsick. While I am encouraged that much is being accomplished in the areas of diagnosis and treatment, hearing the words *you have cancer* makes me feel sorrowful for those who are forced to make this journey.

Cancer is just evil. I have no doubt that it comes from the devil, as the devil's mission is to destroy and dismantle lives. Evil creeps around and rears its ugly head when least expected and leaves feelings of despair, doubt, hopelessness, anger, disbelief. It turns life upside down. When evil invades, the security once known is gone in an instant, leaving fear and total uncertainty. Life is never the same when evil strikes.

Living two doors down put me in a position to be able to help when needed. Words at times fail in this area, so DOING is my job. Her daughter was only 15 when my friend was diagnosed, and there are many things during this stage of a teenager's life that a mother is involved in. I have tried to be attentive to those things while being very mindful that she still has a mother. It is an interesting balance at times. I would never do anything to disrespect my friend, nor do I want her daughter to feel I am attempting to take her mother's place. I have watched her daughter take on

IT HELPS
THE FAN AS
MUCH AS THE
SICK AND THE
CAREGIVER
WHEN YOU LET
FANS HELP.

such responsibility and be forced to grow up nearly overnight. That has been very heartbreaking, as I know her mother would be devastated if she knew all the things her daughter has navigated without her, along with what she has missed. With the loss of short-term memory, the fact that she is unaware is a strange area of gratitude. It's one of the few things I am thankful for about her cancer.

Her husband has been amazing. He is a take-charge, incredibly organized kind of man. He is not the type to ask for any help and makes it all look so easy, though I know it is not. I honestly don't think I have ever heard him complain, not even once, during the last three years. Her husband is very private, so I make every effort to respect that. He is so good at running their home and pays attention to every detail. He cares for her in the same way, thinking of every absolute thing. I believe he takes great pride in being able to provide for his wife and care for their daughter while on this cancer journey. I think it helps him deal with it all in some ways. I say all of this to draw a bit of a picture of my friend and her family. Each family dealing with cancer has different needs and wants. As team members, we have to love and encourage them, putting their needs before ours. I think we have to remember it is about them, not us.

As a bystander, I became the accessory and the embellishment. To be the accessory is to be one who gives assistance and aids in any area. To be an embellishment is to bring joy and help to shine a light in the darkness. I do what things I can, like cooking meals, sending notes of encouragement, silly texts, etc.

I know the most important thing I can do daily is pray. Since prayers aren't often answered immediately or in the time frame or the way we want, we don't always feel like praying is enough. Acts of service are more gratifying, but nothing is more important than prayer for those and their families who are battling cancer.

God has provided in ways that only He could, and I see His mercies each day. While His ways are not my ways and I certainly don't understand most things, I know His will is perfect and that He is taking care of my friend and her family even during this valley.

With that being said, I will continue to be the best accessory and best embellishment I can be. I will follow God's lead and look for His guidance. When I do this, He gives me nudges, when necessary, that help me in fulfilling my role during this journey.

WE'RE NOT FANS. WE'RE DIRECTIONERS. WE'RE NOT OBSESSED. WE'RE DEDICATED. WE'RE NOT FRIENDS. WE'RE FAMILY.

Alone

Some patients are very lucky to have a support system; however, some patients aren't so lucky. So, what if you are alone?

First, let me say you are never alone through this journey. You always have the Lord with you. Second, you have your team of doctors and nurses. It is their job to be there for you and with you. They can be the compassionate person at your side during times of worry or fear. So, if your support system doesn't make up a whole football team, no worries.

If you fall into this category, we have some information to help you. A cancer diagnosis can be overwhelming, so we want to provide you with a way to get the extra assistance you need.

Most treatment centers have social workers or resource personnel on staff. Just what is a social worker

And just as you want men to do to you, you also do to them likewise.

Luke 6:31

or resource personnel? They help you and your family cope with problems that may arise during your illness. They work diligently to make the experience go smoothly. They know most of the answers to your questions, and if they don't, they know how to find the answers.

When you arrive for your initial appointment or treatment, ask if they have a social worker, resource personnel, or a resource center. It is through these resources that you will be able to find answers and cancer resource and educational material. Some offices may even have portable DVD players where you can watch patient education videos. These videos will let you know what to expect with certain treatments.

Treatment centers have information, assistance and resources in most of the following:

- Transportation
- Financial aid
- Emotional counseling assistance
- Nutritional assistance
- Housing
- Programs that give you information on what to expect during treatment
- Massage therapy programs
- Support groups
- Wigs, hats, scarves, and apparel
- Referral services for other cancer needs such as breast prosthesis, mastectomy bras, etc.
- Survivor resources, retreats

If the cancer treatment center doesn't have what you are looking for, ASK! For example, some cancer treatment centers have gas vouchers, but you have to ask for them. Don't be shy about asking. You have to be forward when you are facing a diagnosis. Remember, right now, it is all about you making the first downs.

Another place to go for assistance is always a church. There are many churches that have programs to help those in need. Churches also have volunteers who are available to help in many areas. Once again, you will never know unless you ask. What is the worst thing that could happen? They may tell you no, but probably if they say no, they will give you directions on where to try next.

Not Alone

Mohamed Bzeek is a local hero in Los Angeles. In 1978, Bzeek came to the U.S. from Libya to study engineering. It was then that he met his wife, Dawn, and became a U.S. citizen.

Before marriage, Dawn was a foster parent. She became a foster parent because she was inspired by her grandparents who had fostered many children. Dawn fell in love with every child. She made sure they had everything they needed.

After marrying, Mohamed and Dawn opened their home to many children and also taught classes on foster parenting. They taught a class at a community college on how to handle a child's illness and death. Dawn was highly regarded as a foster mother by many doctors and policymakers. She was part of many taskforces that improved the foster care system.

After taking care of many foster children, Dawn suffered powerful seizures that would leave her weak. The frustrations of her illness wore on her, and in 2014 Dawn passed away.

Mohamed continued to take care of children. He began taking care of terminally ill children who were alone. No one wants to take care of children who are critically ill. These children are sometimes abandoned or born to parents with drug addictions. They have no one, but they now have Mohamed.

Last year Mohamed found out he had colon cancer. He had to have surgery. He had no one. Mohamed stated in an interview that it was terrifying being alone. He thought about all the kids he had taken care of and the children he will take care of in the future. He said, "If I am an adult, 62 years old, and I feel this—that I am alone, I am scared—and nobody tells me it's okay, and it will be fine, I can't imagine how children feel. This experience has humbled me."

Mohamed's experience made him even more empathetic of those children who are alone. With him, they aren't alone. They have a kind-hearted gentle giant to take care of them and love them.

7.
THE TRICKPLAY

Convicts vs. Catholics, the game between Miami and Notre Dame—Lou Holtz vs. Jimmy Johnson. A scuffle broke out before the competition even began. It was going to be a tough one with two riled-up teams.

The teams were finally led into the locker rooms to prepare. "It was quiet," one of the players of Notre Dame stated. Holtz was very calm and said a few words about the scuffle and then ended by saying, "You leave Jimmy Johnson to me." The team was fired up and ready to hit the field.

Back and forth went the game. Notre Dame was up in the first quarter; Miami took the lead in the second; it was neck and neck. Notre Dame scored in the third quarter, which put them on top, but then Miami came back in the fourth to make the game 31–30.

Holtz made two statements that hold true in many situations, whether it's a football game or the game of cancer: One, never underestimate your enemy, and two, expect the unexpected.

Coming back from halftime with Miami up 24–14, Holtz knew he had to do something. He was aware that Notre Dame couldn't beat Miami straight up, so he was going to have to use a trick play.

What was Holtz going to do? He was going to give the ball to someone unexpected—Pat Eilers, a transfer from Yale wearing the unlucky #13. The Yale coach had told Eilers he would never play, but Pat was going to prove him wrong.

Holtz was going to run a play that Notre Dame had never run. Pat got the ball and ran it straight in for a touchdown. Although the ballgame wasn't over, if it had not been for the trick play, Notre Dame wouldn't have scored. Trick plays can win ballgames!

NUTRITION AND THE TRICK PLAY

Trick plays aren't just for football; they are also helpful when you are dealing with cancer treatment. Nutrition can play a vital role in winning the cancer game, but appetite, weight gain or loss, and change in taste have to be taken into consideration. Just how does eating right fight cancer?

Trying to eat healthy during cancer treatment can help you feel better and stay stronger. Take into consideration that there could probably be a cookbook written for every type of cancer, every type of treatment, and every type of person. No two individuals are alike, so what tastes good to one may not taste good to another. Nutrition is an individual game, one that takes lots of trial and error.

When you first visit your cancer treatment center, ask if they have a nutritionist. This person can help you along this journey by giving advice on eating right and maintaining a healthy weight.

Another idea, what I would call my favorite, is to purchase the cookbook *The Cancer Fighting Kitchen* by Rebecca Katz. She gives explanations for just about anything you want to know about eating and cancer. I was so thrilled about her book that I emailed her. She emailed me back the same day.

In her cookbook, Rebecca explains exactly why nutrition is complicated when you have cancer. I'm sure you have heard of people not being able to eat because things taste funny. Rebecca says that your taste buds go kaflooey; however, the technical term is transient taste change. She also explains how cancer therapies can not only damage taste buds or throw them off balance, but they can also cause sudden sensitivity to hot and cold. The good news is that many of these changes wax and wane even between treatments, and they often disappear after treatment. Her book is fabulous; you will want to own it.

Let's talk about these taste buds for a minute. Katz explains that our taste buds have four tastes: sweet, sour, bitter, and salty. Our food mixes with saliva, the taste is sent to the brain, and we react with yum or yuk. When a patient is undergoing treatment, Yuk tends to be the usual reaction. Foods tend to taste too sweet, salty, sour, or bitter because many cancer-fighting drugs also cause the cells in our taste buds to change. Don't panic yet; not all patients experience taste change. There are many different types of chemotherapy drugs, and not all of them affect the taste buds. Some, though, may cause a bitter taste, some a sweeter taste, and some a metallic taste. Some taste may change due to nausea. These changes can happen quickly and stay with you, or they may only last hours. Remember, every drug is different, every person is different, and every treatment is different, so you never know.

So whether you eat or drink or whatever you do, do it all for the glory of God.

1 Corinthians 10:31

127

Rebecca also has a tool to help revitalize your taste buds called FASS, which stands for fat, acid, salt, and sweet. She uses F–olive oil, A–lemons, S–sea salt, and S–Grade B organic maple syrup. FASS fixes troubled taste buds in the following ways: If you have a metallic taste, add sweetener, like maple syrup and squeeze of lemon. If the taste is too sweet, add lemon or lime juice. If the tastes are too salty, add lemon juice. If too bitter, add sweetener, like maple syrup. If things taste like cardboard, add more sea salt. There are also many tips in this cookbook about such matters as difficulty swallowing and dealing with mouth sores.

A third possibility is to find someone you know who understands nutrition. One of my childhood friends, Nancy, is a professor at the University of Arkansas. Her journey began several years ago when she owned a small business where she cooked weekly meals for people. Several of her clients had special dietary needs. Some had diabetes, some HIV, some were children who were obese, and others were undergoing treatments for cancer. Her goal was to keep them healthy and eating.

One of our hometown friends, Stacey, was one of her clients. Stacey had been diagnosed with breast cancer, and the cancer treatments had changed her appetite drastically. Not only was she trying to eat, but she also had a husband and three small children, and they had to eat also. She had many friends who started bringing them food, most of which Stacey couldn't eat. It was great to have meals for her family, but Stacey needed nutrition also. Nancy came to the rescue!

When an oncology patient is going through treatments, many are sensitive to smells, and foods have a metallic taste. This leads to a kitchen nightmare.

It was through our friend Stacey and the cancer season of her life that Nancy learned information about cancer and nutrition. Nancy would use trick plays in the kitchen, adding this and that, trying to alter the taste so it would taste good to Stacey.

Stacey craved salads and fruity foods. Because of the fruit craving, Nancy made a cold strawberry soup. Nancy said, "Yes, it sounds awful, but it was something that Stacey could eat." Weird yes, but it worked.

Because of this, Nancy decided to go back to school and get a degree in dietetics. She continued in school and received her master's degree in human nutrition. She has participated in research studies with cancer patients. Nancy and her colleagues interviewed patients who were undergoing chemotherapy or had gone through chemotherapy or radiation therapy, hoping to find a way to improve mealtimes for them. She took the research and began using trick plays on the taste buds.

Many times, when you fool the taste buds, you prepare foods the patient isn't familiar with. There is no expectation as to what the taste should be because it is an unfamiliar food. As Nancy and I visited over the past several months, she shared her kitchen knowledge with me. I asked if she would write down ten tips for the cancer patient about nutrition.

Nancy's Nutrition Tips

- Not all cancers or treatments for cancers are the same. Just as all people are different, how they react to treatments will differ. You need to find out what works best for you. Most of the people we interviewed were sensitive to smells, the temperature of foods, spices, and seasonings. Most could not tolerate protein foods, such as meat, fish, and poultry.

- Ask your physician for a referral to a registered dietitian nutritionist, preferably one who specializes in oncology. They have seen it all and have a lot of tips on maintaining nutritional status throughout your treatments. Don't find nutritionists on your own. In many states, people may call themselves nutritionists and yet not have any formal training in nutrition, much less a college degree in dietetics. Registered dietitians have, at a minimum, a bachelor of science degree in nutrition from an accredited program, have completed an internship, and passed the registration examination. They have the education and credentials and are licensed.

- If someone is offering to help, don't be afraid to ask for what you need. Several of the patients stated that when people offered to bring food, they wanted it for their family, not for themselves. If you are sensitive to smells, it may be better if the volunteer cooks it at their home and delivers it, where it can be reheated in the microwave. Asking for help with chores you normally do for your family is a great way for someone who does not cook to be involved. If you need help with housework, laundry, or even dog walking, do not hesitate to ask. People want to help.

- Do not start supplements—vitamins/minerals, protein powders, herbal remedies, etc.—without first consulting with your physician or registered dietitian nutritionist. The FDA does NOT regulate supplements. The quality and quantity of ingredients can vary significantly. Many supplements interact with the chemotherapy medications, and some help reduce the severe side effects. You may need a supplement, but let your doctor prescribe it.

- What is considered a healthy diet for most people may not be what is best for you at this time. Depending on the type of cancer you have, your body's use of protein, fats, and carbohydrates may be affected. Your body may not be able to absorb the nutrients from food. Work with your dietitian or physician to help with these issues.

- Don't believe everything you read on the Internet. Find credible websites when searching for information, like eatright.org, or the websites of organizations like the American Cancer Society, Mayo Clinic, MD Anderson, the Academy of Nutrition and Dietetics. Now is not the time to risk your health, so trust sources that have the research to back the information.

- It is important that side effects that affect eating and weight loss be treated early. Your doctor can prescribe medicine to increase appetite, treat nausea and vomiting, treat and prevent mouth sores, and pain. Dry mouth is a common side effect, and the patients I've interviewed suggested Jolly Ranchers. Also, try to keep a water bottle with you as often as possible.

- Protein foods are difficult for most oncology patients. A complete protein, such as meat, chicken, and fish, provides the essential amino acids your body needs to grow and repair. But meat is not your only protein option. Eggs, dairy, and cheese are excellent sources of complete proteins. Combining grains, seeds, and legumes can accomplish this protein need. Common pairings are beans and rice, bread and peanut butter, hummus (which is made of chickpeas) and wheat bread or crackers. There are many possibilities, and vegetarian cookbooks are an excellent source of recipes.

- Rest. Take care of yourself. It's okay if you can't do the things you used to. Save your strength to fight this horrible disease. That is the most important aspect.

- Prevention is the best way to outwit cancer, but sometimes you can do everything you think is right and still get that horrible diagnosis. If this happens to you, take the time to learn about cancer prevention, for your specific diagnosis. When you have finished treatments and are able, include these lifestyle interventions to promote improvement in diet and exercise. Your goal is maintaining a cancer-free life.

My next tip is to turn to people you know who have been through treatment. The Chemosabe Women's group gave me insight to treatment 101. I sent them all a questionnaire, and they began jotting info down.

- If metallic taste, add fruit to your water; lemons or oranges seem to work better.
- Lemon drops or jolly ranchers help/Russell Stover lemon drops (cuts metal taste).
- Drink lots of water. Drink smart water.
- Eat when you can to keep your strength up.
- Get in your protein (peanut butter, eggs, beans).
- Use plastic utensils.
- Eat things you have never eaten; you won't expect the taste before you taste it.
- Marinate meat in different things you have never tried—fruit juice, sweet or sour sauces.
- Stay away from bad odors.
- Choose foods that smell good and taste good to you.
- Cold or frozen food is better than hot.
- Flavor foods with spices you usually don't use.
- Eat organic.
- Non-GMO foods.
- There are excellent nutritional books out there to help cancer patients.
- Have a nutritionist develop a diet for you.
- Read ingredient labels, and try to eat protein, fruits, vegetables.
- Protein shakes.
- Drink lots of Gatorade and PowerAde.
- Treat yourself with food at times.
- B complete vitamins.

- There are plenty of drugs to help with nausea, so don't hesitate to ask your doctor for what you need.
- Listen to your body.
- Phenergan (helps with nausea).

There is no magic wand to wave and know what to eat and what not to eat. You must remember everyone is different, every treatment is different, and all taste buds are different. Try new things, throw in a trick play, and eat something you have no idea how it is going to taste. Trick plays usually win.

Remember these six key points that the National Cancer Institute gives us in the article "Overview of Nutrition in Cancer Care."

- Good nutrition is important for cancer patients.
- Healthy eating habits are important during cancer treatment.
- Cancer can change the way the body uses food.
- Cancer and cancer treatments may affect nutrition.
- Malnutrition can happen in cancer patients.
- It is important to treat weight loss caused by cancer and its treatments.

You can be healthy with cancer. You will have good days and bad days, but don't give up on food. Use the trick plays and try new tastes. It is simply by trial and error. If you don't like it, don't eat it.

Nutrition is something that depends on the type of cancer you have and the treatment you endure. Our son-in-law, who has esophageal cancer, could only eat soft food and liquids. With him being 6'6" and losing down to 180 pounds, it gets to the point you don't care what they eat. You just want them to eat so they will gain weight. Our brother-in-law, who had brain cancer, only craved sweets. You do what you need to do to keep a healthy weight; that is your primary goal.

Let food be thy medicine and medicine be thy food.

Hippocrates

Read about Kris Carr

In 2003, Kris Carr was diagnosed with incurable cancer. Doctors gave her seven months to live. Kris states on her website that even though she can't be cured, she can be healthy. She turned to her garden and her kitchen, which she calls her pharmacies, to create food that would help her be the healthiest she could be. Good nutrition can create a healthy and energized body and mind. You can fight cancer with your fork. Kris has written several books, many that deal with diet. Follow the link to read about Kris and order her nutritionally filled books: www.kriscarr.com.

Personal Essay

Whole Health

April
Cancer Patient, Wife, Mom, Dietician

To look at her, you see only beauty and good health, but little do you know that on the inside lives cancer. For 17 years, she has been dealing with the demon that lives in her gut. Since 22, she has had surgery after surgery and kept her cancer at bay with a chemo pill.

When asked what she thought contributed to her being so healthy, she stated that it is "WHOLE HEALTH." You can't just take one piece of being healthy to live with cancer; you have to have the whole body. Physical, mental, spiritual, along with a well-balanced diet and exercise.

Being a dietician, she eats well-balanced meals and tries to stay away from processed foods. She integrates many foods in and out of her diet. She said, "You need to eat as people ate years ago. From the garden and from animals that you know are clean eaters themselves." She stays away from soft drinks and drinks kombucha. "Now and then you can't help but eat junk," she said, "but I don't eat junk very often."

When asked what she thought causes cancer to mutate, she stated that some cancers are genetic and some are environmental. It just takes one thing for cancer cells to go haywire. She's not quite sure what she thinks about diet contributing to cancer growth. You can find pros and cons for different types of diet. It may be diet, and it may not diet. There would need to be research done with every different situation. However, she did say that she feels much better when she eats healthy. One thing that can be 100% sure of is that her way of eating and keeping the whole health attitude has kept her alive with cancer.

Whole health—having alignment in all areas of life so that the outcome will be optimal healing. When you have "whole health," you will be able to live healthy with cancer.

HANDLE IT

Mike
Prostate Cancer Patient and
Father of Breast Cancer Patient

We were heartbroken. It is one thing for a parent to be given a diagnosis, but for a child to hear those words is unthinkable. I had been diagnosed with prostate cancer, had the robotic removal, and had clean scans. My daughter, however, was a different story. At the age of 24, when most young women are beginning a new season of their lives, our daughter learned she had breast cancer.

How do you handle when your child is diagnosed?

My wife and I knew the strain that cancer puts on you. Cancer to us was evil, invasive, painful, and emotional. We knew, however, that we were going to get through our second bout with cancer by leaning on our faith. The best way to handle cancer is with daily prayer. My wife and I prayed every day. Sometimes we would just pray and then at other times we would pray and cry.

Even though the diagnosis was trying, we were able to see the glass half full because of our daughter. It was easy for us to stay positive because our daughter was positive. She began writing a blog sharing her experiences. Her friends drew near keeping her motivated. Her boyfriend did what he could to make every day joyful.

Everyone worked together as a team doing their part to help us push through.

We knew that it was easier to fight cancer when you are well rested, eating well, and exercising as much as you could. My wife read ingredient labels and cooked food that was healthy. We ate more protein, fruits, and vegetables and pushed through the carb cravings. Every day there was some type of yoga or walking that was done. The exercise may not have been executed at a fast pace, but we were up and moving.

Our daughter, even though fighting cancer, made our environment a happy one. Our home found joy through cancer because we knew how powerful God is. He is bigger and stronger than any cancer.

Now that my daughter and I are both in remission and she is to be married, we pray every day for cancer to disappear from our lives. We know that every day is a gift, and we tackle each day with a twinkle in our smiles. We appreciate every little thing in life. If cancer returns we will once again give it to God to handle. He can handle it!

PERSONAL ESSAY

A Must

Misti and Lauren

When you get your list of medications and treatments to fight cancer, nutrition should be on the list. Good nutrition during and after cancer is part of the treatment plan.

You need a dietician. This professional is a vital part of your team. Many cancer patients struggle with weight loss, decreased appetite, and taste change. A dietician will make sure you meet the goals for calorie intake, protein intake, and fluid intake. You may only

138

need to meet with them once, but it could be the one person that could save your life.

A dietician is going to keep you as healthy as possible during your treatment. Depending on the type of cancer and its treatment, you may find food and eating to be a battle. A dietician can provide suggestions on the easiest way for you to consume calories based on the challenges you are facing. Their job is to help you maintain a healthy weight and to assist in other needs such as supplements, nutritional counseling, feeding tubes, poor appetite, and nausea.

After our son-in-law completed all of his treatment, no one told him about what he should and shouldn't eat. After going through a treatment regimen of chemotherapy and radiation that was followed by the removal of part of his stomach and esophagus, you would think someone would have said, "This is what you should and shouldn't eat."

Fast forward one year and two months. Scans were done, and two lymph nodes and the surgery spot lit up. After two scans, an EGD was done with biopsies taken. A week later, the pathology report showed no signs of cancer at the surgery site. So, what about the lymph nodes? Because there is so much inflammation at the surgery site due to the food he had eaten, they had to wait eight more weeks for more scans to see if the lymph nodes were just reactive due to the inflammation of the esophagus. All of this could have been avoided if someone had sent him to a dietician.

A dietician is an essential part of the cancer team.

8.
PROTECTIVE EQUIPMENT

On November 28, 2013, the Pittsburgh Steelers faced their rivals, the Baltimore Ravens. The Steelers had the ball second and goal, the score Steelers 14 to Ravens 22. Only 1:26 left in the fourth quarter. The ball was snapped, and running back Le'Veon Bell was handed the ball. Bell dove in head first to attempt a touchdown. As Bell was charging in, three Ravens blocked him. There was a collision and helmet-to-helmet contact. Bell's helmet flew off. No protection was there between him and everything around him. Bell left the field injured, and the touchdown was no good.

All football players must wear helmets and other protective gear to reduce the chance of injury. The jersey shows the player's identity, but it also keeps shoulder pads in place. The helmet and the facemask are designed to protect a player's face and head from serious injury. Some players may wear other protective caps on the inside of the helmet for added protection. Most players also wear mouth guards to protect their teeth. Pads on different parts of the player's body are there to absorb the physical blows to shoulders, sternum, rotator cuffs, thighs, elbows, hips, tail, and knees. Players also wear cleated shoes for protection and stability.

Several committees work diligently to review injury data and examine videos to see how the injuries occur and then to figure out ways to prevent the injury. We know that wearing protective gear does help, but it doesn't prevent players from getting injured.

Knowing you are playing a high-speed, impact sport requires you to think before you step foot onto the field. Players must ask themselves, "Am I protected?" The players must realize that something may occur even though they are equipped with the proper equipment.

> Finally, be strong in the Lord and in his mighty power. Put on the full armor of God, so that you can take your stand against the devil's schemes. For our struggle is not against flesh and blood, but against the rulers, against the authorities, against the powers of this dark world and against the spiritual forces of evil in the heavenly realms. Therefore put on the full armor of God, so that when the day of evil comes, you may be able to stand your ground, and after you have done everything, to stand. Stand firm then, with the belt of truth buckled around your waist, with the breastplate of righteousness in place, and with your feet fitted with the readiness that comes from the gospel of peace. In addition to all this, take up the shield of faith, with which you can extinguish all the flaming arrows of the evil one. Take the helmet of salvation and the sword of the Spirit, which is the word of God. And pray in the Spirit on all occasions with all kinds of prayers and requests. With this in mind, be alert and always keep on praying for all the Lord's people.

> Ephesians 6:10-18

All I can do is
put on my
armor and
brace for the
arrows.

Jamie Kennedy

INSURANCE PROTECTION

Just as athletes wear protective gear to protect them from the hits on the field, we need protection for the game of life. The protection we need during this life game is health insurance for illness.

Some people wonder why we have to have this protection. When athletes step onto the playing field, they don't plan on getting hurt, but just in case, they put on all their protective gear. During many games, no one receives an injury, but they are still prepared with the protection they need. We don't expect nor do we want to get sick, but it does happen. The last thing anyone needs to worry about when dealing with cancer are the bills they acquire.

Insurance policies protect us from major medical expenses such as doctor's visits and surgical procedures in the event of the unexpected. Many different insurance companies offer a variety of policies. You will pay less for covered in-network health care on most health policies, even before you meet your deductible.

Insurance policies, statements, and everything that goes with the financial end of medical expenses can be tough to understand. Even educated people don't always understand the fine print. The best thing you can do, on the front end of the diagnosis, is to visit with the financial person at your cancer center or doctor's office. Then find someone outside the medical facility to help. Visit your insurance agent or find a friend who works in the insurance business. You can also visit websites with information on insurance.

If you have Medicare or Medicaid, you will find that these two entities have different rules and regulations.

142

- Medicare is the federal health insurance program for people who are 65 or older, certain younger people with disabilities, and people with end-stage renal disease (permanent kidney failure requiring dialysis or a transplant, sometimes called ESRD). Go to this website to read more about Medicare: www.medicare.gov.

- Medicaid is a jointly funded, federal-state health insurance program for low-income and needy people. It covers children; the aged, blind, and/or disabled; and other people who are eligible to receive federally assisted income maintenance payments. Read more about Medicaid here: www.ssa.gov/disabilityresearch/wi/medicaid.htm

If you qualify for either of the above, you will need to check with your medical facility to see what is covered.

When my daughter's husband was diagnosed with cancer, she knew the bills were going to roll in. Her husband had great insurance with the school district and a secondary disability policy with another company; however, she didn't know any of the details that went with these coverages. My daughter knew she needed help, so she called one of our family friends, Kelsi, and began asking questions. Kelsi invited Lauren to come to the office where she spent two hours explaining what she should do and what she shouldn't do, what to pay and what not to pay, how to read the medical statements, and what had been paid or pending. This made it much easier. Now, every week Lauren sits down and goes through all the bills and knows what to do.

May the perfect grace and eternal love of Christ our Lord be our never-failing protection and help.

Saint Ignatius

When my sister-in-law's husband was diagnosed with cancer, one of her best friends worked for an insurance company. She volunteered to go through everything for her.

I turned to these two insurance women for help while writing this chapter. Below are some helpful tips from both of these ladies.

INSURANCE 101

Know your health plan. All carriers are required to make a summary of benefits of coverage (SBC) readily available to you. This SBC will contain all the information you will need to know about your annual maximum out-of-pocket, copays, deductibles, etc.

First things first: Talk to your local agent who should be there to help you. The last thing you need to worry about is insurance when dealing with your diagnosis. Your local agent will be able to help you understand your benefits in detail and assist you in sorting out bills and figuring out what is covered. Let your local agent bring you the peace of mind you need regarding insurance so you can stay focused on what is most important.

When the bills start coming, a good rule of thumb is to wait at least 30 days or until the second statement comes before you begin payment. This gives the provider and insurance carrier time to make sure everything was coded and filed accurately. You always want to match your bill with your Explanation of Benefits or Personal Health Statement. Below is an example of what could happen:

You may have received a bill from the hospital for the total amount charged by your doctor, which in this case would be $448.00. However, if you look further you will see you were discounted by insurance, and the carrier paid towards your bill. In reality, you would only owe $30, which you will see in the furthermost column under total. You will want to make sure that the $30 on your personal health statement matches the bill from the doctor before you pay the bill.

INSURANCE TIPS AND TRICKS

1. **If you can find someone in your family or a close friend who understands insurance** and would be willing to handle your insurance/medical bills, ask them to assist or even to manage these bills for you. If you do not have anyone knowledgeable about insurance, visit the business office at your cancer center. Cancer centers usually have personnel who will help you with your insurance needs and questions. These people are called case managers, and they will study your case. If that isn't an option, go directly to your insurance company.

2. **Create a "fact sheet"** to include full patient name, date of birth, social security number, home address, insurance policy information (including phone numbers and where claims are mailed). If a spouse is the policyholder, please include date of birth, social security number, full name. Include all information identifying patient and policyholder. If someone were assisting, they would also need a copy of this. It should be considered confidential and handled as such.

3. **Power of attorney:** If you are the patient, you might check with a lawyer to sign a power of attorney or other legal document giving the representative permission to discuss your medical bills with the providers. Many times, accounting departments for medical facilities/providers will not discuss a patient's medical bills without authorization from the patient. *Check with an attorney about the proper paperwork needed.*

4. **Folders:** It is very hard to keep bills in a "monthly" folder as the dates of service span many months. Keep an easily identifiable folder with all medical bills and explanation of benefits (EOBs) in one spot where they are readily available. If you have someone assisting you, bundle your bills and deliver to them. Your representative will keep up with everything.

5. **Explanation of Benefits (EOBs):** An EOB is what you will receive from the insurance company showing what the company paid on the medical bill. When you receive EOBs in the mail, compare the date of service on the EOB to the appropriate medical bill. Bind these documents together. Once claims are filed with the insurance company, paid by insurance, and you have paid the balance, file the paperwork in a paid folder. Mark your folders with the contents (i.e. paid, pending, etc.). If your representative is handling for you, consider giving them signed checks so they can pay balances when EOBs are received.

6. **Always make sure** you have received an EOB from the insurance company before paying the bill.

7. **If you get** a form asking for additional information, complete as soon as possible. Most of the time, the company will not process the claim until you return the completed form.

8. **You might receive a bill** from a provider, and it does not show that insurance has been filed. You will need to call the number on the bill and make sure they have the insurance information. Have your information handy so you can give it to them.

9. **Anytime you speak with someone** at a provider's office, document who you spoke with and when (date, time). Document the action taken (or that will be taken). If they are going to file the claim with insurance, simply make a note to that effect. If they are going to rebill the claim, note that also. ALWAYS write down the name of person and the date you spoke with them.

10. **Your insurance company may refuse to pay** for treatment. If this happens, do not take NO for an answer. Call and keeping calling your insurance company. Talk to your doctor. Call the company that develops the drug. Don't stop. Call your legislators. Talk to anyone and everyone.

DISABILITY INSURANCE

If you have worked and paid into Social Security, then you may be able to receive SSDI (Social Security disability income). This is available when an illness keeps a patient from working. It is a process. The patient must fill out an application and must meet Social

Security's strict definition of disability in order to qualify for SSDI. If at first you don't get approved, you can reapply and appeal. For more info, visit this link: www.cancer.org/treatment/finding-and-paying-for-treatment/understanding-health-insurance/health-insurance-options/social-security-disability-income-for-people-with-cancer.html.

OTHER PROTECTION

Other things need protection. Life does go on, and things still have to be done even though you or a loved one is sick. One of my friends who is a cancer survivor stated this fact that is so true: "In spite of illness or tragedy, you still have to take out the garbage and pay the bills."

If you are away from home for an extended period and you have obligations such as young children, utility, and other bills, etc., you will probably need to call on others for help. Included in the *Scouting Report* are sheets for you to record all of your information. It is simple enough that you can hand the information page to whomever and ask them to handle things for you. This is not a time when you need to have your electricity shut off, your life insurance lapse, or your kids left at school.

I WILL HANDLE IT

Amelia, Fan

"I will handle your medical bills." Words I spoke to one of my dearest friends within a matter of days after her husband was diagnosed with brain cancer. Working in the medical industry all of my adult life, I knew the amount of effort (physically and mentally) needed to keep up with medical bills, insurance EOB's, etc. I knew this would and should be one less burdensome challenge she needed to deal with.

I believe through personal experience that there are many different ways you can support people during difficult times and that God makes sure all of the right people are in your life during these times. There are those who bring food, wash your car, and pick up people at the airport, whatever the need during a tough situation. I am blessed to be the one to help ease this burden of busy paperwork, numerous (duplicate) bills, overpayments, and phone calls. I'm thankful that God chose me to love His precious family in this special way. Being allowed to take an unnecessary burden from them warms my heart.

NO TIME TO WAIT

For two months, he had been living with prostate and bone cancer. He was ready to get the show on the road; however, insurance had become an issue. For over 70 years he had been paying for insurance. He had never been sick; this was the first time he needed the insurance policy. He began every day calling the same number trying to get some results only to hear the same answer, "No you have not been approved." A person can only take so many no's—especially when you are waiting to begin treatment for cancer. After many calls, he finally told the insurance company, "The next phone call you get will be from my lawyer." Out the blue, insurance decided to approve treatment. The wait time was finally over.

OUT OF NETWORK

After our son-in-law's surgery for esophageal cancer, the bills began to pour in. In the stack was a huge anesthesia bill. What is this? Insurance had not paid on the anesthesia bill at all. Lauren called and began to ask questions. She finally got an answer, "Well ma'am, the anesthesiologist was out of network, so your insurance won't pay." The hospital was in network, the doctors were in network, but the anesthesiologist was not in network. When the anesthesiologist walks in the room to prepare you for surgery, you don't ask, "Excuse me are you under network?" Wouldn't you think if everyone else in the hospital who is working on you and the hospital itself is under network that the anesthesiologist would be? After several persistent phone calls, insurance said they would pay.

SMALL PRINT

He knew something was not right. Strange things had happened. His wife's brain was not functioning the way it should. They went to the doctor, and all that was going on was documented. What they needed was

150

a brain scan. Insurance said there were not enough symptoms to pay for the scan. After several visits and calls, insurance still said, "No Scan!"

He didn't know what to do next, then the Lord spoke. The Lord said, "Look at the small print." He began reading through their insurance policy. In the policy in small print, it stated that if the patient is taken to the emergency room, a scan can be performed without preapproval and it will be paid.

The next morning, he returned to the clinic. They still said no to the scan. Insurance had not approved payment. He argued, and they finally said," Sir, take her to the ER!" That is what he did, and the scan was performed.

Just what he thought, brain cancer! Thank goodness for the small print.

PERSISTENCE

The only surgeon who would perform the type of surgery I needed for my cancer was located out of state. Insurance told me to find someone in state. There was no one! There was not a specialized surgeon in our state who performed the surgery I needed. I began to call everyone I knew who could help. I researched. I called legislators. I wrote letters. I appealed the insurance company. After being persistent, I received approval from my insurance company to have the surgery 1,450 miles away.

9.
FOURTH QUARTER

The seniors of the 1964 Arkansas Razorback football team had decided to dedicate themselves to doing whatever it required to earn success on the field. Their decision shaped the course of Razorback football history. One game after another the Razorbacks became more determined. When they weren't named national champions by several outlets, they headed into the 1965 Cotton Bowl Classic. They decided all they wanted was a perfect season 11–0.

In the first quarter of the Cotton Bowl, the Razorbacks jumped to a 3-0 lead, but Nebraska responded with a touchdown in the second quarter, breaking Arkansas's five-game shutout streak. The score remained the same until the fourth quarter when Arkansas mounted an 80-yard drive, which led to a touchdown with a successful extra point. This score led to a victory and a perfect season.

As we are coming to the end of our playbook, we want to remind you that it isn't over until the completion of the fourth quarter. The fourth quarter is crucial in this game of life. As Frank Broyles said to his 1964 undefeated Razorback team, there is no substitute for the preparation of the fourth quarter. You must be prepared to play your best before the fourth quarter begins.

We have to look at the cancer journey like this also. When you get to the fourth quarter, you are probably going to be more tired, you are probably not going to be as strong, you are probably going to be beat up, and you are probably going to be discouraged— BUT now isn't the time to quit. The fourth quarter is when you gather it all up, put all your fight out there, and give it your all.

Just like the Razorback team of 1964, you are a champion. You are prepared, and you are ready for this game. You may not have been named the national champion, but you are a champion. WE together are going to change the landscape of cancer forever!

Coming Back Strong

Peyton Manning is noted as being one of the greatest athletes of all time. He is also known to have made an incredible comeback after he underwent multiple neck surgeries along with spinal fusion surgery. These surgeries forced him to sit out an entire year. There was talk that he would never return to the playing field. Manning wasn't going to let these setbacks interfere with his playing career. He dismissed all that everyone was saying and began rehab. He worked extremely hard and by the end of the season was throwing passes again. After the injury, the Colts cut Manning, but he signed on with the Denver Broncos. Many sports commentators didn't think Manning could come back strong from such setbacks. He did have his challenges, but he quickly returned to his old form. His return was in 2012, in which he did well, but the following year he shattered offensive records. He threw for 5,477 yards and 55 touchdowns. Manning's recovery is one of the most significant ones in NFL history. He continued and sealed his comeback with a Super Bowl win in 2016.

GET MOVING

During the fourth quarter, after your cancer regimen, you will be ready to go through the recovery process. It will take some time to bounce back. Your body has been through a trauma, and it needs to be babied back to health. To begin, you must approach the post treatment slowly. Even though beginning at a slower pace, don't ever give up. Cancer may have limited you, but you can and will get back on the playing field. Remember the body is an incredible machine that God created. Now it is time to get moving physically, mentally, and spiritually.

PHYSICAL

It is a known fact that the body is an amazing machine that can come back from severe trauma. When you are ready to come back physically, you have to remember that your body has been through a difficult time. You may have limitations that you didn't have before cancer. To have a successful physical comeback, you must adapt to the changes that have taken place. You can't change anything that has happened, so you need to find a way to accept and move forward.

CHANGING POSITIONS

After cancer treatment, some decisions have to be made. You must ask yourself three questions:

- Am I willing to get back on the field?
- Am I willing to change positions?
- Am I willing to listen to the coach?

I sat down with a friend who is a personal trainer to get first-hand information on how cancer patients can get back on the field. Here are her thoughts:

- A patient must understand that they have been down. They have had an injury on the field, and it will be a gradual process to get back on the field of play. Getting back in shape is 99% a mental game. The mind will tell us many things, but our bodies are magnificent machines that God created, and He created us to do more than we think we can. Assess where you are on the field and then accept where you are. You may have been a linebacker before cancer, but now you have changed positions to be a receiver.

- Getting back into shape is an individual task. That is why these professionals are called PERSONAL trainers. They personalize on the person as an individual. Every patient's cancer was different just like their treatment was different; therefore, their exercise program will be different. You need to answer these questions before getting started:
  ≈   What was I like before cancer?
  ≈   How did cancer affect me?

155

You can
throw in the
towel, or you
can use it to
wipe the
sweat off
your face and
keep going.

≈ Where do I want to go with this exercise program?

≈ How can a trainer help me?

- It is imperative before you begin a fitness regimen that you talk with your doctor. Find out exactly what you can do and what you can't do. What part of your body do you need to be careful with? What would cause more harm than good?

- For the trainer to do their best work, you need to be honest. You need to say what hurts and what doesn't. If you aren't honest with your body, then you may cause more injury, which can lead to more limitations.

- Diet is very important. Diet is to the body what gas is to a car. A car can't run on bad gas. A body can't get back into shape on bad food. With cancer and because of treatments, it may take time for food to taste good again. Diets can be tricky; however, a proper diet is essential to working out the body. Lots of protein is needed. Due to your muscle not being used, you have probably lost muscle. Protein will rebuild your muscle.

- According to the American Cancer Society, it is vital for cancer survivors to regain strength and rebuild tissue by eating a healthy diet. A diet that is full of fruits and vegetables is recommended, along with one that includes plenty of high-fiber foods. They also recommend limiting red meat intake.

- Check and recheck your mental game. When you begin your exercise program after cancer, it is like

156

you are going into the ballgame 21 points behind. You aren't going to win with one touchdown. To have a comeback, it has to be one play at a time, pushing slowly and gradually. You are starting in the other team's end zone and not physically where you used to be.

- Listen to your trainer and don't put limitations on yourself. As humans, we tend to think we can't do it. When you are frustrated and have been hit over and over again, you tend to sit on the bench. You usually do what your mind tells you you can do and not actually what you can do. See yourself in a different position. See yourself moving forward and regaining the strength you once had.

YOU HAVE SETBACKS IN YOUR LIFE AND ADVERSITY. YOU CAN BE DISCOURAGED BY IT OR HAVE THE COURAGE TO GET THROUGH IT AND BE BETTER.

TIME AND EXERCISE

In addition to what is listed above, Brian Hodge offers in his article "The Rule of Two: Coming Back after Injury" a useful rule on exercise. If you experience no pain during or after the exercise, add two minutes to your next regimen. As long as your body feels sound, add two minutes of exercise. However, if you experience unfavorable symptoms, subtract two minutes from your next exercise regimen. Do not increase your time until you have at least two consecutive successful training sessions.

OTHER THINGS TO REMEMBER AFTER TREATMENT

FATIGUE

Most cancer patients suffer from fatigue—loss of energy. If you have fatigue, be sure to speak to your physician about it. It is a good idea to tell your doctor anything you are feeling. There may be an underlying cause that you don't understand.

If you have days when you have a loss of energy, it is a good idea not to do strenuous exercising but go on a short walk. Being tired can take a toll on the body. It can lead to muscle weakness. This is why it is important to get back physically active as soon as you can. There are advantages of being active after treatment.

MENTALLY

Cancer leaves a mark, even when you are given a clean bill of health. When beginning the journey of life after cancer, you need to understand that everyone is different. No one's comeback is going to be exactly like that of another cancer patient. Just as each cancer diagnosis is different, so is the journey back to health. The comeback also takes time. One must be given space and support to talk about it. You can't be rushed to "move on." Moving on can be gradually balanced while recognizing there is new life and things that aren't cancer-related. Cancer has changed your life, your habits, your days, and your nights. Cancer has become your normal. Therefore, you have to find a new normal after cancer. This new normal

158

can't be forced. When pushed to move on too quickly, a person will be robbed of strong feelings that need to be brought to the surface.

Life after cancer can also be frustrating. You have been benched, and you have had to change positions. You may have been a receiver, but you have changed into a lineman. Changing positions and being placed on the line has caused you to be hit over and over again. With that, you must get a new mentality. The mindset of getting back is a gradual process. You cannot start where you left off because your body has been through some tough plays.

Every day a person experiences thousands of thoughts. Those thoughts can be positive, but they can also be negative. There are common feelings that are the same with everyone.

One thought that many patients have is the fear of the cancer returning. Patients begin to live from scan to scan, having what people call scanxiety. One friend told me that the day she receives the results of the scans are the best days, then she goes back to fear. Thoughts will creep in every day that makes her worry.

Feelings of fear and reoccurrence are normal. All cancer patients feel this way. As time goes on, those feelings get less and less. Find activities that take your mind away from cancer. When fear creeps in, lean on others for strength; cry if you need to. You are very vulnerable, and that is okay.

How do you live not in fear? The first thing is faith. You have to trust in the Lord. Go to him daily and ask for continued healing. The second is always have follow-up appointments. You and your doctor know your body and when things are normal and when they

But those who hope in the Lord will renew their strength. They will soar on wings like eagles; they will run and not grow weary, they will walk and not be faint.

Isaiah 40:31

159

aren't. The next is to be healthy. Eating clean will help your body work the way it should and rid your body of toxins. Exercise is great for the brain and your thoughts. By exercising you reduce stress and tension. Feeding your body nutritionally and working on your body with exercise is not only good for you, but it will also help you recover from the cancer treatment.

Another part of the mental recovery is realizing that your body has changed. You may have weight gain or loss. You may have insomnia, or you may need to sleep more. Racing heartbeat, dry mouth, headaches, or aches and pains may occur. Many of these things are caused by the treatment that your body endured.

Survivor's Guilt

Besides having emotions such as joy, fear, relief, and gratitude, there is also the nagging feeling of guilt. Being a survivor makes you ask the question why? Why did I survive and someone else did not? This is very normal. Survivor's guilt is not only familiar with cancer patients, it is common with those who have been involved in war, natural disasters, or even accidents. One of the best ways to move past the guilt is to talk about it. Another way is to look ahead and do something good out of the experience. Be the survivor who uses your experience to be productive and fruitful.

There is nothing wrong with seeking professional help for the mental part of after cancer. Mental health is just as important as your physical health. A counselor can help you with the emotions you are having. He or she can help you to let go of thoughts that are holding you back from living a productive cancer-free life.

CHEMO BRAIN

Research has shown that one in four people with cancer report memory and attention problems after chemotherapy. Chemo patients call this chemo brain. Chemo brain is a real issue. Chemo brain may last a short time or may go on for years.

Just what is chemo brain? Chemo brain causes the patient to have trouble concentrating, remembering details, or multi-tasking. It also cause patients to forget things that are usually no trouble recalling, to take longer to finish things, and to have trouble remembering common words. Most of these short-term problems get better as the underlying problem is treated. To help with chemo brain, the patient should get enough rest, exercise, eat properly, keep a calendar of events, and ask for help if needed. Read more about chemo brain here: www.cancer.org/treatment/treat-ments-and-side-effects/physical-side-effects/changes-in-mood-or-thinking/chemo-brain.html.

SCARS

We are all wounded. Some wounds are hidden, but yet some are visible. These scars are a reminder that you have survived. When you have a unique scar, a scar you are proud of, you want to show it off. Some scars though, such as cancer scars, you want to tuck away. You want to hide the scar and never be reminded of where you got the scar. It can be difficult to be proud of the scar, but the scar shows to the world that you are a survivor. Scars give others hope. Scars tell your story.

We all have scars, but scars don't define us. Scars don't limit us. Scars if anything expand us. People all over the world are searching for others who have the same scars they do.

Scars make us ask, "Why did this happen?" We must change the question to, "God, what do you want me to do with my scars?"

Ultimately the choice is yours as to what you do with your scar. You can either propel yourself to something greater than your scar or let the scar hold you back. Your choice. Make the best decision.

SPIRITUALITY

When things are going great in our lives, it is easy to have faith and believe in God. When the tables turn, and things aren't going well, we tend to have emotions against God. With many things of this world, we have questions that haven't been answered and many questions that will never have an answer. Dr. James Dobson said once, "To try to understand God's ways is like an amoeba trying to understand how the human body works. We just can't do it." So true!

People may say to you, "Why would God have given you this illness?"

First, God didn't give you anything. God is equally sad when bad things happen to us. Going with that statement, we have to remember that God is good and that He uses things for the good. The best thing we can do is look to Jesus to reconnect or keep connected with our faith. When we think of what Jesus did in all circumstances and situations, we will be put at ease. Think about it: Jesus grieved over the brokenness of the world, he wept over death, and he was sad when there was a sickness.

162

Cancer is the reminder of how our world is: broken. Sins of the flesh have caused our world to be spiraling out of control. It is what the flesh has done that is the culprit of many things that bring us sorrow. It is absolutely not God.

With that being said, I do want to say that you can be filled with anger. You can get mad at God just as fast as you can pray to God. God knows how you feel, and He can take your anger. Remember he weeps when you weep. God gets it.

Many questions will never be answered on earth. God heals some, and some have eternal healing. We will never know the answer "why?"

There are some things I do know. God loves us, He will heal us, and He has a restored world for us.

The hardest thing to do is trust and believe. Now is the time that you dive into the word of God. His word is the truth, and His word leads you to peace. You must understand that everything is for good and God does have a purpose for what you endure.

Therefore, if anyone is in Christ, the new creation has come: The old has gone, and the new is here!

2 Corinthians 5:17

The Other Side

When the treatment is over and the cancer is gone, many people will be excited for you, and then they will move on. People go on about their lives as normal, but you, on the other hand, will be reminded of the change daily. This will fade as you move. You have a new you—you after cancer. The old self is gone, and you have stepped into your new life.

There are parts of this "new self" that are okay. One is that it is okay to let go of those who don't understand the new you. You don't want to waste time. Move forward making the most of every minute of every day. You won't sweat the small things anymore because you truly know the difference in big and small.

To look at cancer through another lens, unlike what others can do, is to appreciate life. Let your passion be your purpose. Let your story spread to others who are taking that first step onto the field with the enemy.

LUCKY

Sarah,
Cancer Survivor, Lymphoma

I had a life ahead of me, but first I was going to deal with cancer. Why? I will never be able to answer that, but it doesn't matter because I am lucky.

Hodgkin's lymphoma—those two words that so many fall prey to. I was in my early 30s and had a regimen of poison ahead of me. Four different chemos every week. These four chemos are referred to as ABVD. ABVD is the most common regimen in the United States to treat Hodgkin's. The red devil was part of ABVD, and it was supposed to be the worse. Two days after chemo I would feel like a brick truck had run over me. My bones would ache so badly that I would just cry. I wore out heating pads from lying on them so often. After the chemo, I received radiation in the Stanford V regimen. Radiation made me more tired than I could ever imagine.

Treatment was the hardest four months of my life, and as bad as it was, I would say it was good. That may seem strange. However, it killed the cancer. It did what it was supposed to do.

Right after I completed my entire cancer regimen, I got married. As women, we want the natural progression of life. We graduate high school, go to college, get married, and then have children. I wanted a life that was normal, or at least what I thought normal was.

A great fertility doctor told me I would probably never have children on my own. He said there was a 10% chance. Within two years of being told that, I found out I was pregnant. Today I have two beautiful baby girls. I am reminded as I look at my two precious angels that only God has and knows the plan for you. Even though doctors know many things, they do not know everything.

One doctor told me I was one of the lucky ones. At first, I didn't understand, but then I learned. If you get a cancer diagnosis and you beat the cancer, you truly have a new outlook and understanding of what is important in life.

If you have been given a bad diagnosis, stay positive and hopeful. You may be lucky like me. I am lucky in more ways than one.

You have searched me, Lord, and you know me.

Psalm 139:1

PERSONAL ESSAY

THE GIANT PAUSE

Lauren, 27,
Caregiver, ER Nurse, MS in Nursing

Life was going as we had planned. Married, working, saving, enjoying days together, then it happened—a giant pause! Someone hit the pause button in the middle of our dance, and it wasn't me. I had no control over whether to play or to stop. Our normal life was now on pause.

That is what happened when cancer came drifting into our lives. Everything we had planned was in pause mode. We went through a year of test after test, treatment after treatment, surgery, more treatment, doctors' appointments, and blood work. You name it, we were in the middle of it. The lyrics of cancer continued. Then we finally came to the end of the song, or was it?

Some think that when you receive your last treatment, have scans, and they are clean that your dance continues, and it does in some ways, but not the way it was playing out. There is a verse after cancer that goes on. It may have a verse and a chorus, or it may just be a chorus, but whatever it maybe, it leaves you with notes that you have a difficult time singing.

Our new dance was just beginning, and we had to learn it step by step.

For a year, our steps will include tests, scans, blood work, and our regular day-to-day routine. There will still be the anxiety after each scan and scope. There will still be days that the cancer treatment will steal my husband's energy. There will still be the days that we are sitting in waiting rooms for the answer that lies behind door number 1,2, or 3.

Even though the treatment is over, the life pause is still lingering over us. We pray every day that the information located on the lines of the reports gives us good news. Good news will allow our play button to stay down and our pause button will no longer be an issue.

A dear friend and co-worker sent me this text:

All throughout the Bible you see God's people, people He loves and adores, waiting—pausing, waiting on Him to change their circumstances. God has ordained waiting to be a master part of His plan. I choose to believe the longer we have to pause and wait for something, the blessing is increased … increased to more than we asked for. Take heart, friend. It's all part of His plan … and I promise, it's better than you have imagined.

We continue to dance just as we have done during each measure. Sometimes we are in step; sometimes we are out of step. We at times are off key, but we continue to push play even during the pause. The pause may have distracted us for a while, but with faith, we will continue to dance through the pause that changed our lives forever.

10.

OVERTIME

November 1, 2003, the University of Arkansas and the University of Kentucky were playing each other. However, the ballgame wasn't over until November 2. At the end of the second quarter, Arkansas was ahead 21–7. After halftime, Kentucky ran onto the field ready for action. Arkansas fumbled, and Kentucky scored. During the fourth quarter, Kentucky tied it up. Overtime was the next place to go. The teams went back and forth for seven overtimes, which set a record for the most overtimes in college history. In the last overtime, Arkansas was able to secure the win when Kentucky fumbled the ball and Arkansas recovered it. At 12:01 November 2, the ball game was officially over with an Arkansas win. The ending score was Arkansas 71–Kentucky 63.

When in overtime, the margin for error is small. One step too soon or one step too late can lead to a loss. Plans have to be made before you step on the field. When the team is prepared, every play will be carried out right on time.

So what do you do when you are in cancer overtime?

You go into overtime with a positive mindset. You step onto the field, and you take every inch around you. You go over each play with your team. You make sure everyone is headed in the same direction. All areas of the game, physically, mentally, and spiritually, have to be up to speed. There is no room for error. You make certain what you need is there, and it is there when you need it. You rehearse in your mind a victory. You play with confidence that you know what the outcome will be. You and your teammates are pros going the extra mile for the win.

Part of recovery may be relapse. Dust yourself off and move forward again.

Steven Adler

RELAPSE

The NCI dictionary defines *relapse* as the return of a disease or the signs and symptoms of a disease after a period of improvement. Relapse also refers to returning to the use of an addictive substance or behavior, such as cigarette smoking.

What happens when there is a relapse? A relapse is a recurrence. It likely occurs because the original cancer cells survived the initial treatment but were too small to be detected during the follow-up. Cancer may come back in the same place, or it may be in a new location. Even when cancer reoccurs, the name given is the primary place the cancer originated. Cancer is more likely to come back if it's fast growing, if it is advanced, or if it is widespread. Most cancer occurs in a typical pattern, and doctors are very familiar with this.

The American Cancer Society lists the three different types of cancer recurrence:

- **Local recurrence** means the cancer has come back in the same place it first started.

- **Regional recurrence** means the cancer has come back in the lymph nodes near the place it first started.

- **Distant recurrence** means the cancer has come back in another part of the body, some distance from where it started (often the lungs, liver, bone, or brain).

The odds of this happening depend on many factors including the type of cancer you had.

Finding your emotions all over the spectrum is normal. You may feel like "Here I go again!"

Here are some questions to ask your physician. These come from an article from CURESEARCH:

- What is the chance this relapse can be cured permanently?
- What is the chance this relapse can be controlled for a period (even if it does not eventually result in cure)?
- What are the standard treatments in this circumstance?
- What role do research options play in this circumstance? Are these available in my treatment center, or would I need to consider traveling elsewhere?
- What are the likely impacts (medical, psychological, social) of each of these options?
- Is it appropriate that palliative care is involved, even if there is still hope for a cure?
- How will we monitor the cancer now?
- Why did this happen?

Cancer is unique to each person, and so is a successful outcome from a relapse for the individual.

Recurrence is the reason why having follow-up check-ups and scans is important. When you are finished with your cancer regimen, you should receive a follow-up care plan. This plan will schedule appointments with your doctors and schedule any other tests that are necessary. Depending on the type of cancer you had, blood work and scans are possible. Your doctor will also tell you what signs and symptoms you should be aware of.

If you feel it is time for a second opinion, get one. This is your life. You have a choice in what you do and what you put your body through.

WINNING IS ALWAYS FUN, BUT WHEN YOU HAVE TO WIN IN OVERTIME, WHERE YOUR PLAYERS HAVE TO GO THAT EXTRA MILE, IT'S REALLY GRATIFYING AND SPECIAL.

Personal Essay

Grateful

Sherry,
Cancer Survivor

Cancer can be lonely and scary, but it was not going to frighten me to death. After my diagnosis, I gathered my team. The RAMS—Right Attitude Makes Sense. I knew I was going to need people praying and fighting this battle of mine. My team consisted of friends, family, and churches throughout the United States. I was thankful for every single one who prayed for me.

In 1982 at the age of 32, I had my first cancer diagnosis of Hodgkin's. Back then there was no social media, so any communication about my health was given over the phone or through the mail. I decided that if The RAMS were going to walk beside me, I needed to let them know how I was doing. After every doctor's appointment and treatment, I would write

171

each member of my team a note giving them an update on my health. Letters not only let them know what was going on, but it was a healthy outlet for me. It kept me going. During my breast cancer in 2008, I was able to use Facebook, so I didn't have to write letters. Writing and journaling kept me positive.

At times during cancer, it's hard to be grateful and thankful. Sometimes you have to look hard to find the positive. During my first diagnosis in the 80s, cancer treatment wasn't as updated as it is today. The medications for nausea didn't work as well. I was sick every two hours on the hour. I tried several medications. Yes, it is hard to be grateful when you are vomiting. However, I did. I thanked God every time I threw up. That might sound crazy, but I thanked Him for giving people the knowledge to develop chemo medication that would save my life.

I AM A SURVIVOR was and still is my theme song. I am surviving. I have survived Hodgkin's and a reoccurrence of it. I have survived breast cancer. I have had heart surgery and also pneumonia that doesn't want to go away—BUT I am grateful. I am thankful that I am a survivor.

PERSONAL ESSAY

SHARING

Sherry,
Cancer Survivor and
Mother of Cancer Patient

Cancer! I was not going to let it dominate me emotionally or spiritually. I was diagnosed with cancer twice in 1991 and once in 2006. In 2006, my diagnosis was grim—Stage 4 metastatic cancer of the internal mammary lymph node. I give all the glory to God for my survival.

Many people shared my illness. My friends and family were by my side every day. My community was incredible. My doctors became not just doctors, but friends. Cards and meals were delivered every day. Prayers were prevalent throughout our community. Friends drove me to radiation. I was amazed at how much support surrounded me.

I have recently been given a new assignment on this earth, and it is linked to cancer. It is not something I have chosen, nor do I want to have to do it as a mother. I learned and pushed through my diagnosis, and now I must share my cancer knowledge with my daughter.

My daughter was diagnosis last year with a squamous cell. It began as anal, then moved to thigh and shoulder, and is now in two lymph nodes. As mothers, we want to share things with our children, but this isn't something I wanted to share with my daughter.

Even though medicine has improved since I had cancer, I have the knowledge to help my daughter through the journey. I understand the fatigue. I know the toll it takes on your body mentally and physically. I know when to help and what needs to be done.

I am thankful that God helped me survive so I can share my strength with my daughter. I share so that she will become a survivor also.

The R words are important and scary in cancer— Recovery, Remission, Relapse

Misti Coker

11.

POSTGAME: THE FIFTH QUARTER

FOR THE PATIENT

Teams don't win all the time. Top ranked teams eventually lose. In 2007, Michigan paid the Appalachian State Mountaineers $400,000 to travel to Ann Arbor to provide the Wolverines a nice win.

With 28 seconds left in the game, Michigan set up for a 37-yard field goal attempt that would likely give them the win. Instead of making the points, the kick was blocked, and ASU walked away with the victory.

Fans probably thought they were reading the score wrong when they saw Appalachian State 34–Michigan 32. This game is listed as one of the top college upsets of all time.

When teams walk onto the field, they know someone is going to win and someone is going to lose. We too walk this field of life understanding the progression from birth to death. I feel with a disease, if terminal, knowing death is ahead leaves families with raw emotions. It helps to prepare for the days ahead.

A year after my dad had survived throat cancer, he was diagnosed with pancreatic cancer. Twenty-two years ago, there wasn't much hope with a pancreatic cancer diagnosis. The oncologist told my dad he had six months to live.

At the time I was 29, I was married with two toddlers, and my third daughter was due in July. My mom and I made the next six months memorable. The girls and I spent every afternoon with my mom and dad. We had many ventures walking around the block, looking at the flowers, and gazing up at the sky. Time passed on, and we knew that the time we had left was limited.

I gave birth to my third daughter, and even though my dad was emaciated, weighing only 120 pounds and standing 6'2", he was there. I gave him the privilege of naming this little bundle of joy. He held Anna every day for the next week until he had to be placed in the hospital.

It was getting closer, and he knew it. One day he looked at me and said, "I need for you to do something for me. Would you go to the house, get my brown suit, and take it to the cleaners? I don't want to be in the casket and smell like mothballs." It was then that we laughed through our tears.

A week later he passed away.

Difficult? Yes, BUT—and there is always that but—my dad was finally healed.

When cancer strikes, there are two ways God heals:

1. He heals on earth
2. He heals in heaven

It is hard for us to see death through God's eyes. We only view it through our eyes. As humans, we are selfish. We want our loved ones to stay here on earth.

This is the day the Lord hath made let us rejoice and be glad in it.

Psalm 118:24

Though his last few weeks were difficult, the time between the diagnosis and the time when Dad was placed in the hospital were full of memories.

I wrote a story once entitled, "The Empty Chair." None of us want an empty chair, but it isn't our choice. God has a plan and a purpose for us, all of us. When a loved one dies, we do have an empty spot in our heart, but we must remember to fill the void with all the memories.

None of these words probably matter right now since you are facing difficulty. During this time, you just need Jesus. I found an article written by Andy Rau, senior manager of content for Bible Gateway:

> My wife and I were driving in the rain and fog. I could barely see anything except for the stripe on the edge of the road and the taillights in front of me. The same goes for tragedy and suffering in our lives. We can't make out all the details, they are obscured from our view, but some Biblical truths illuminate some points for us. As we follow these lights of truth, they will lead us in the right direction and give us some understanding.
>
> God is not the creator of evil and suffering.
>
> Though suffering isn't good, God can use it to accomplish good.
>
> The day is coming when suffering will cease, and God will judge evil.
>
> Our suffering will pale in comparison to what God has in store for his followers.
>
> We decide whether to turn bitter or turn to God for peace and courage.

So yes, cancer sucks and remember it's not over until the fat lady sings. Don't let her start singing yet. Don't ever give up even if you have gotten a terminal diagnosis. Everyone on earth is terminal, and only

God knows when our departure will be. Take time making memories, memories that will last a lifetime. **And remember this: Miracles DO happen! You may be a miracle!**

How Do I Prepare?

For the Patient and the Caregiver

There is somewhat of a blessing in knowing you are terminally ill. You may think this sounds bizarre, but it is the truth. I have experienced death both ways. I knew my father was going to die, but my sister died suddenly. There is something to be said about being able to tell your loved one how you feel. Sharing with them your thoughts and them sharing their thoughts with you. With my sister, none of us got to express anything to her. There are many things I would've liked to have said.

Will this preparation for death be easy? No, but it will be worth it for our loved ones left on earth.

There are many emotions that one will experience while preparing for death. Sorrow, anxiety, anger, acceptance, depression, and denial are the normal feelings. These emotions can be present in the patient and the caregiver.

When preparing for this day, talking about it will help, but it can be difficult to be led into the conversation.

How do you begin?

Approach the topic gently. Ask questions that will lead into the discussion. For example, you can ask:

What do you worry about? How can I help? Is there anything you want to talk about?

You may want to bring in a preacher, a doctor, or a counselor to help with the discussion.

One of the most important points to remember is this, "Timing is everything." If the discussion doesn't seem to be comfortable or flowing in the right direction, stop. It may not be a good time to talk about the situation. Wait for a better opportunity.

Besides the emotional side to dying there is also the practical side that involves such things as life insurance, living wills, power of attorney, and DNRs.

You need to check to make sure you have a copy of your life insurance and that it is up to date and nothing is due. Your loved ones need to know where it is and who carries your policy.

The living will, power of attorney, and DNRs are important because they carry out the patient's health wishes during the end of life. A living will is a written document where the patient has listed what they want medically done if they become mentally or physically unable to make decisions. A power of attorney is a form that designates a person to act on the patient's behalf when necessary. A lawyer takes care of both of these items. These items should be completed in advance. Links to these forms can be found online or obtained at a lawyer's office. When you have the forms filled out completely, give copies to your physician and your family.

DNR stands for Do Not Resuscitate. A DNR instructs medical personnel not to use equipment that would restart the heart or use equipment that would artificially breathe for the patient. A DNR is a form signed by the patient that states that if the heart stops, the patient does not want medical personnel to revive them. Even though the patient has a DNR, that doesn't mean medical staff will not be there. The patient would be made comfortable and be allowed to have a natural death. If there is not a DNR, the medical staff must work on the body to try to revive it. A DNR form may be included in a living will or advance directive. A living will is a legal document that lets people state their wishes for end-of-life medical care.

DNR forms are simple to prepare. They are usually just one-page documents. Different states have different laws for such legal documents, so you want to make sure your DNR complies with the state where you are living. Not just those with a terminal illness or at risk for medical problems should have a DNR. Anyone who feels strongly about not being resuscitated or intubated should consider having a DNR in place.

It is best to have multiple copies of all forms on file to share with family and medical personal. If you do not have the monetary funds to get these forms completed, there are ways to get this accomplished. Certain law firms will do things *pro bono*. Pro bono means they will do work without payment. Some law schools offer services at no charge because their law students need practice. Ask at your cancer center or doctor's office if they know of anyone who will do these things for free. Usually, a social worker can find a place for you. You may also want to check with your county or state bar association. There is also a Pro Bono website—www.probono.net/oppsguide/—that

God saw you getting tired, and a cure was not to be. So, he put his arms around you and whispered, "Come to me."

Author Unknown

helps the disadvantaged. You go to the website, choose the state where you live, click find, and a list of lawyers will pop up that will produce these forms at no charge.

No one is ever prepared for death. No one ever wants the end to get here, but it makes the process easier having these things completed.

Remember we were not created for this world of chaos. God wanted us to live in a sin-free world, but in the beginning, that was changed and sin occurred. What one must do is make the best of the earth while they are here, but be prepared for the eternal home. The eternal home is better than the world we live in today.

WHAT IF WE LOSE?

FOR THE CAREGIVER

Marian Dickson Ruffin is one of the dearest, sweetest Christian women I know. I grew up spending time at her home with her daughter. Marian's husband, Dale, was diagnosed in 2002 with cancer. He passed away in 2003. Marian was familiar with death, not only personally, but also because she and her husband owned a funeral home. For years, they served the community during loved ones' most difficult times.

In February of 2003, Marian was driving her husband to chemotherapy. It was a cold, icy, and drizzling wet day. She recalls how she began to cry. She was mad. She was angry at God because of cancer. She told her husband that God could have healed him. Dale told her, "Our knowledge is so limited, but God's wisdom is so much greater. We have had a blessed marriage. You work through the anger and trust in God. You have to trust in Him."

180

For a year, Marian dealt with her grief and sorrow. She knew that God works everything for good. Even though Marian had prepared herself for Dale's death, she wasn't ready. You may think you are ready, but you aren't ever prepared for death. Death is final, and when death occurs, you know that you won't see your loved one anymore.

After a year, Marian decided she was going to begin a GriefShare group in our small community. GriefShare is a non-denominational faith-based group. Those in GriefShare are caring people who are willing to walk alongside you through one of life's most painful experiences. GriefShare enables you not to have to walk through the grieving process alone.

Marian was already a servant of the Lord, but because of Dale's death, she became an even larger servant. Because of her decision to gain something positive out of death, she has lead hundreds of people through the grief process. She has now been teaching GriefShare for 13 years through her church.

I visited with Marian and asked her to share a few key points about grief and GriefShare.

One of the most important pieces of GriefShare is the acronym **DEER**:

D=Drink Water (Drinking water will keep your body hydrated. Your body needs to be well hydrated to function properly.)

E=Exercise (Exercise is good for your mental and physical health.)

E=Eat (Don't forget to eat. You need good, clean food to keep your body nourished.)

R=Rest (Get a good night's rest.)

When you die, it does not mean you lose to cancer. You beat cancer ... by how you live, why you live and the manner in, which you live.

Stuart Scott

WHEN SOMEONE
YOU LOVE
BECOMES A
MEMORY, THE
MEMORY
BECOMES A
TREASURE.

OTHER INFORMATION ON GRIEF

- Grieving is normal and necessary

- When we lose someone, we do grieve, everyone grieves, but no one person does it the same way.

- It is impossible not to grieve. If you try to ignore grieving, you will be like a tea kettle holding in the steam, but then reaching the boiling point and exploding.

- You can't go around grief. There is no shortcut, and there is no perfect way.

- Talking is necessary. Telling your story is a great way to walk through your grief.

- Men have the mentality that big men don't cry, but men need to cry and grieve just as women do.

- The worse times can lead to the best times if you allow it.

- Grief is messy. It is not orderly. There is no certain order of the stages of grief.

- You can be in more than one stage of grief at a time.

- When grieving, a person will be like a tangled ball of emotions.

- Be in the present. Think good concrete ideas.

- Try to stay in a positive mindset.

- Do breathing exercises.

- Always be prepared to DO THE NEXT THING. Don't get stuck.

- Don't make any major decisions for a year.

- Write what is called a grief letter to your family and friends. (Go here to see a GriefShare example session: www.griefshare.org/downloads/gs/samples/ Workbook_Sample.pdf

- Make a scrapbook of memories.

- Have a get-together with friends/family to share memories of your loved one.

Grief is not a sign of weakness nor a lack of faith. It is the price of love.

Unknown

One of the best decisions you can make if you are dealing with the death of a loved one is to find a GriefShare group. GriefShare is worldwide, and there are hundreds of support groups. You can go to grief-share.org to find a GriefShare group meeting near you.

Anticipatory Death

Anticipatory death is a real thing. If your loved one has been sick for a very long time and you are the caregiver, you may grieve before death takes place. When you become aware that death is coming, anticipatory death will likely occur.

Anticipatory death can carry many of the same characteristics as grieving after death. You can be angry, sad, depressed, and forgetful. You can also isolate yourself. As with grief after death, there is no right or wrong way to grieve, and no two people go through anticipatory grief the same.

At times during this grief process, it will be somewhat of a relief when your loved one does pass. You know and understand that your loved one is in a much better place and is pain-free. However, this can

Do not let your hearts be troubled. You believe in God; believe also in me. My Father's house has many rooms; if that were not so, would I have told you that I am going there to prepare a place for you?

John 14:1–2

lead to a feeling of guilt. You need to remember that even though there is somewhat of a relief, it doesn't mean you didn't love your loved one any less. This reaction is normal, especially under a situation that is stressful and overwhelming.

All of this is normal. You have to remember to take care of you, find a support group, and say yes to counseling.

Hospice

When the patient gets to the end, hospice may be called in. What is hospice and what do they do?

Hospice began years ago as a shelter for tired and ill religious pilgrims. Hospice is available to you 24 hours a day, seven days a week. The hospice team is made up of doctors, nurses, social workers, and clergy. They give you physical, emotional, and spiritual care. This can take place in your home, nursing home, or assisted living center. Hospice works with the patient and the family devising a plan. They participate in a variety of daily tasks. Hospice is usually covered by insurance and may also be covered by Medicare and-or Medicaid. There may be some out-of-pocket expenses.

When my neighbor was dying, hospice came in. Summer was the hospice nurse's name. She was the sweetest person. She was caring and empathetic. She knew what to say and when to say it. She knew when to help and when to back off. She let Lynn, the care-giver, do as much or as little as he wanted. She was there at any time day and night. She was present until the very end. She did her job and did it well. She was there in all aspects of the dying process.

184

PRE-PLANNING

Earth has no sorrow that heaven can't heal.

Thomas More

Death is inevitable for all of us. It makes it easier on your loved ones if you have planned for your departure from this world. One of my best friends owns a funeral home, and they, like many other funeral homes, can help a person plan.

Planning gives the family the opportunity to express their wishes and feelings openly in a personal manner. A carefully pre-planned service can be the most comforting to the family, as it spares them from having to face decisions that are emotionally difficult.

Funeral homes have a trained funeral director who can help you make important decisions. Planning also makes financial sense. Funerals can be costly, and being on a payment plan will also save your family extra expense.

The funeral home in our town has a website and offers a funeral checklist. This checklist provides a list of information and items the funeral home will need. These things need to be taken with you when you meet with the funeral director.

- Full Legal Name
- Home Address
- Social Security Number
- Date of Birth
- Place of Birth
- Father's Name
- Mother's Maiden Name
- Veteran's Discharge Papers (DD-214)
- Recent Photograph
- Highest Education

- Occupation
- Place of Burial (if applicable)
- Clothing
- Clergy Name and Phone Number
- Survivors (name and relationship)
- Insurance Policies (if applicable)

In the *Scouting Report*, you will find this information in a table form to be checked off when you gather what is needed.

WHAT DO I DO?

FOR THE CHEERLEADER OR THE FAN

We had been friends for years. We lived across the street from each other. I had been a friend of the husband since our younger days. Our children were the same age, and they had grown up together. We celebrated together and cried together. There were no secrets amongst all of us. We all shared life.

In 2015, Natalie was diagnosed with triple negative breast cancer. She was brave, and she fought it. She was in remission in November of that year. It was a wonderful few months. Then in January, she had a recurrence. It was back in her lungs. For months, she struggled. At the end of April, it had spread to her brain. There was nothing they could do.

For several weeks, we pitched in. We cooked, cleaned, and washed clothes. We did anything we could think of to make the next few weeks comfortable for their family. The weekend before her death, a dear childhood friend, Amy, came to visit. There wasn't anything we could do. The two of us grabbed some blankets and sat on my neighbor's front porch in the swing. We were

186

there all day and into the night. We were there if anyone needed anything, but we were out of the way. We were the buffer. We were there to run interference. If anyone came to visit, we took a message or we would text my friend and ask if he wanted company. Throughout the day, he would come out to visit and take a break. We didn't do much of anything, and it didn't matter. What mattered the most was just our presence.

It is often difficult for friends to be placed in a death situation. It is awkward and uncomfortable. What you need to remember as a friend is this: At times nothing matters but your presence. When someone is suffering from death, the person usually doesn't remember what you said to them anyway.

When placed in this situation, here are some tips to follow:

- Ministry of Presence—Just being present is often enough.
- Sometimes NO WORDS are best.
- There are no magic words.
- Listen more than you talk.
- Choose words wisely (understand that you can't fix this).
- Just help. Do the little things you see that need to be done—gathering the trash, for example.
- Do not say, "Call me if you need anything"— because they won't.
- Share memories.
- Love your friend. Just show up.
- Follow your friend's lead; grief is a personal experience.
- Check in after weeks and months have gone by.

Create in me a pure heart, O God, and renew a steadfast spirit within me. Do not cast me from your presence or take your Holy Spirit from me. Restore to me the joy of your salvation and grant me a willing spirit, to sustain me.

Psalm 51:10–12

*For we know
that if the
earthly tent we
live in is
destroyed, we
have a building
from God, an
eternal house in
heaven, not
built by human
hands.*

2 Corinthians 5:1

WHEN WE ASK WHY

God's purpose and plan
Is sometimes concealed,
But someday His purpose
Will be revealed.

Someday God's wisdom
Will make it very plain
Why problems were permitted
And how He uses pain.

Things thought illogical—
Disease, tragedy, fear—
Will someday make sense
When God makes all things clear.

We'll see the Lord's purpose
From the Lord's point of view,
And we'll know the answers
In ways we never knew.

Until we're home with God
Some answers must wait.
Until His plan unfolds
We're called to live by faith.

Perry Tanksley

188

THE BLESSING

Marlo,
Age 12 when her mother died
of breast cancer, now 50

No one ever thinks of death as a blessing, but the day my grandfather (Papa) joined his Holy Father in heaven blessed me abundantly.

Papa was a Godly man who for over 50 years had led the choir and the congregational music at his church. He shared his love for music with his daughters, Carol and Nancy. They called themselves THE INSPIRATIONS, and that they were. They traveled sharing their testimonies and their talents with many churches. The word of God would lift off their lips during their speaking and their singing.

When my Papa died, my aunt, Nancy, wanted to play a song of him singing "The Old Rugged Cross." She handed me the tapes and said, "Please find Papa singing 'The Old Rugged Cross.'" As I was driving home, I began to listen to the tapes. One song after another bellowed from my speakers. Then came the blessing. It was her. It was Carol, my mother. I heard her voice. She was on the cassette giving her testimony. She was explaining what God had done for her even though she was fighting cancer. She thanked God for giving her some time with her daughters. She thanked Him for allowing her to share her testimony.

I had not heard my mother's voice since 1979. Over 30 years since I had heard the sweet sound that used to take care of me. I began calling everyone who loved my mom and turned my speakers up to full

Sometimes by losing a battle, you find a new way to win the war.

Donald Trump

189

I believe that whatever comes at a particular time is a blessing from God.

A.R. Rahman

volume. Her voice took over my car. I shared her voice with my husband and my sons. They were able to hear what my mother sounded like.

As I visit with my friends about her voice, tears fill my eyes. God blessed me that day. He knew I needed a wink from Him. My Papa is now in heaven making heavenly sounds with his daughter. I on earth am still today listening to the blessing that overflows my ears with joy.

PERSONAL ESSAY

SOLVE THE PUZZLE

Fan

The time had come. No more meal trains, no more motivational gifts. Over. It was the end. We had all been there. Anything they needed.

At the last appointment, they had learned that cancer had spread. From breast to the lung, now to the brain. Her family asked, "How long?" You never know. Her body was young, only 40. She was strong. It was going to take a while for her body to shut down.

They got her home and made her comfortable. The shutting down of her body began. We all watched. It was a slow process. It was like a preparation.

No, we didn't want her to pass. However, we knew her quality of life was gone.

Hospice was called. They were kind and attentive. They weren't pushy, never in the way. They were there to help when needed. They became part of the family, just like many of us did.

190

Neighbors, that is what we were. Every day I would drive by and see her getting her mail. The sweetest young lady I knew. She would smile and wave. Ten years younger than me and married to one of my best friends. The years that I knew her, I never heard her speak a bad word about anything. She was a true southern young lady. We both had a love for pizza and *Wheel of Fortune*. Many nights, I would ride my bike over, and we would watch trying to solve the puzzle.

For 17 days, we watched and waited. We saw her body deteriorate. One thing after another began to shut down.

May 17, 6:30 p.m. I will never forget. Her husband and sons had gone to the high school sports banquet. Only she and her dad were there. It was with him, the man who protected her during her 40 years of life, that she took her last breath. She knew he was the only one who could handle it.

Looking across the street, I saw them all rush in. I knew. I could feel it. She was gone. No more pain, no more medication, no more waiting.

The cancer puzzle everyone had tried to solve. Medication after medication, treatment after treatment, but only God could solve the puzzle, and that he did. My friend was at peace in her Father's arms. The hardest piece of the puzzle had been placed, and it was finished—solved.

He will wipe every tear from their eyes. There will be no more death or mourning or crying or pain, for the old order of things has passed away.

Revelation 21:4

THE RIDE

Kim,
Daughter, Caregiver

> *What a caterpillar calls the end of the world the master calls a butterfly.*
>
> Richard Back

I've heard it said, "We are all just a phone call away from our knees." My call came on June 18, 2012. Cancer had decided my dad would be his next stop. The "Demon," as I like to refer to cancer, introduced himself and made it entirely clear we were in for a "Ride." His name was Multiple Myeloma, translated to me as Bone Cancer.

Clearly unfamiliar with his name, the room began to spin and I thought is this the ride he spoke of? Or could this type of cancer be like a merry-go-round? What if it was like a roller coaster or bumper cars. Am I going to be bungee jumping? Without any warning, I found out it was going to be all of the above and then some.

Cancer has no agenda, and rules do not apply. Cancer can go along for months or years just as smooth as a merry-go-round, toss you around like a roller coaster, beat you up like bumper cars, and leave you screaming as you spiral out of control, not knowing if or when your feet will ever hit the ground, as if you were bungee jumping. As I began learning to deal with this demon as a caregiver, I felt as if somehow my life had become a permanent "Severe Weather Advisory." Conditions were always favorable for a severe outbreak at any given time. I found myself going through so many emotions, and then panic set in.

The days ahead were very frightening. Daddy would undergo reconstructive surgery on his broken leg and then be given a team of doctors to handle his case. His team consisted of an oncologist, heart specialist, ortho specialist, and kidney specialist, and one doctor could not make a move without the consent of the others. Daddy's hospital stay would last 24 days, and during that time I was informed I would be the main caregiver since I lived in the same town. Now keep in mind, I have three sisters—two are nurses and one really not capable of this task—and then there was ME ... a high school graduate with only a "Life Lesson" degree!!

My daddy had a saying for people when he thought they didn't know what they were doing; he would say, "It's obvious they only have a fifth-grade education." As I found myself surrounded by a team of doctors explaining things to me every day, I am not ashamed to admit I became one of those with a fifth-grade education, but oddly enough, Daddy didn't see me that way. I had become his eyes, his ears, and his feet. Between the two of us, we were determined to make this work. Somehow, someway, we were going to learn to live with cancer and not let it beat us down.

Over the course of the next four years, we found ourselves back in the hospital multiple times, and each time we did a little better. I was learning to communicate with my dad on a whole new level. Our roles reversed. I was now the provider for who used to be my provider. It was difficult at first, this is my dad, but when I finally realized he wasn't comfortable being in charge, it became my duty.

The years ahead were challenging for us both; we had both lost our lives as we once knew them to be. Daddy was unable to drive; he couldn't wear his regular boots, and walking to the mailbox was a challenge. Eventually, the walks stopped, too. Then there was me; I was a wife, mother, grandmother, and his kid. Didn't anyone understand I have a life, too? I didn't sign up for this. I didn't want the well-being of my dad in my hands!

There were days I didn't want to get out of bed, and there were many nights I drank myself to sleep. My expectations from others were overwhelming me and angered me from the lack of help. I was rolling in a self-pity party of one! Then it happened. Daddy called. He had a surprise and wanted me to come out and see it. Dreading yet another trip to the country, I went out, and there he sat in his recliner grinning from ear to ear. I asked what's up? He just sat there still grinning, and then I saw it. After two years, he finally managed to put his boots on and could walk in them! He was as proud as a young child who just learned to tie his shoes! At that moment with tears in our eyes and smiles on both of our faces, we realized we did it! We were living with cancer and growing together! I wasn't his caregiver, his daughter, or the boss. I was his "teammate," and he was mine! Through all his struggles, he finally accomplished a part of his past life, before cancer! At that moment, I realized how something so small in our lives could become something so amazing. I knew then we were going to be okay.

I decided if I did not have any expectations from others, I would never be disappointed. That day was a victory for Daddy, and oddly enough in the months and years to come, we started seeing and appreciating any other little success that came along. I'm sure they were always there, but we just didn't know how to find them—but we did now.

Daddy would have several other breaks through-out the years, and like most cancer patients, chemo is usually involved. I remember his first day of chemo. I was scared, and I know he was too, but he would never admit it.

BE SOMEONE'S SUNSHINE WHEN THEIR SKIES ARE GRAY.

The staff, nurses, and doctor were very welcoming and made us both feel very comfortable. Eventually, Daddy made friends and enjoyed his weekly chemo buddies. They all sat on the same row for years; I called them the "boys of cell block C." February 2016, cancer took its toll on cell block C, and Daddy found himself the last one on the block. After that, Daddy chose never to sit on that row again. That was a sad day for us both; we realized what once was his comfort zone had become a tainted memory. Cell block C had become Death Row.

On June 19, 2016, I spent the afternoon with Daddy; it was Father's Day. We talked about every-thing except cancer; it was a good day! On June 20, 2016, cancer called again, only this time Daddy was not responding.

I found myself once again spinning. Just when I thought I understood cancer, I found myself on that roller coaster! On June 27, I was told by his doctor that there was nothing more that could be done. Hospice was called in on June 29. Once again, I found myself talking with someone I didn't know and not understanding what she was saying or what I was about to do. She went over several questions, and I can honestly say I don't remember any of them except for the very last one. In the most calming, sweet, caring voice, this lady that I had only met 45 minutes earlier looked at me and said,

"Which funeral home will you be using?" At that moment sitting in the hospital cafe, I have never felt so lifeless. I remember asking, "You don't think he will be going home?"

On June 30, hospice was coming for Daddy; I remember asking God to give me a sign that I was doing the right thing. I walked into Daddy's room, and he did not know who I was! I was enraged! After all we had been through, that was it? I was furious with God; how could he do this to me? It wasn't until now as I write this that I realized this was the best thing God could have done for us both. You see, if I had seen any improvement in Daddy's condition, I would stop hospice, and God knew this. He knew he needed to go to extremes to save us both! Daddy passed away July 4, 2016, at 3:55 p.m.

It's been eight months since Daddy passed away. I am still learning a new normal. Life as I knew it will never be the same. I can't pick up where I left off because I'm not the same person anymore and I don't want to be that person. Cancer truly changed my life. I thought at the time it was the worst thing ever, but now I'm grateful, I'm stronger, I've learned to listen to silence, and I still try to find those small victories every day.

My arms feel empty from time to time, but they are much stronger. My heart aches, but it has found compassion.

For those of you who find yourself as a caregiver, pray and give it all to God. He's in control and will never give you more than you can handle. Caregiving is terrifying and rewarding all in one. No question is a dumb question. Get to know your health providers, and don't be afraid to speak out. In some cases you are speaking for the patient. There are many health providers out there for home care as well. Utilize them from therapy to home health medical care. Know you are never alone! Laugh, smile, and talk a lot, but most important *listen!* Never say never! Be proud of what you are doing; not everyone can take on this position. Everything happens for a reason, and something positive always comes from the negative.

I will be forever changed. Cancer and I have a love/hate relationship, and I am forever bonded to it. Cancer handed me grief that is unexplainable and love as I've never experienced. It humbles all those around it; it truly teaches you your life is a gift.

Strangely, cancer gave me my daddy back. Life is so fast and furious that we forget to slow down, and those around us are affected by it. Daddy and I reconnected in a way I would have never imagined. We laughed, cried, argued, and we learned so much from each other, and there were never too many I love yous along the way.

I spent the afternoon the other day with a young man whose father is facing terminal cancer, and I can see the stress in his eyes. He is now holding the title of caregiver, and I feel there is nothing I can do but listen and be an example for him. He received a phone call that afternoon that his dad needed to go to the emergency room. The look in his eyes was too familiar, but he too will make it through, and he will never walk in life the same, and for some reason, I find comfort in that, and he will too one day.

Be shepherds of God's flock that is under your care, watching over them—not because you must, but because you are willing, as God wants you to be; not pursuing dishonest gain, but eager to serve; not lording it over those entrusted to you, but being examples to the flock. And when the Chief Shepherd appears, you will receive the crown of glory that will never fade away.

1 Peter 5:2–4

Sometimes the things that take the most give the most.

Misti P. Coker

Cancer took a lot from my daddy, but in the end, it made this very large man who was always outspoken, a little rough around the edges, and sometimes a little scary, and turned him into my Gentle Giant. For that, I will always be grateful!

And in the END… NO REGRETS!

12.

THE FOREVER CHEERLEADER

There are no regrets in life, just lessons.

Jennifer Aniston

Greg Murtha was a Razorback cheerleader in the 80s. He had a smile you would never forget. Even after he retired his uniform, he was still a cheerleader. His personality enabled him to be a part of many adventures in the business world. Greg joined the iDonate team and served as president, head of marketing and sales, and chief connections officer. He also launched Leading with a Limp, a nonprofit organization to serve as the home base for his personal ministry.

Greg's toughest ball game began in 2011. At 46 and in the best physical shape, his life was interrupted. Five words changed his life: "Mr. Murtha, you have cancer." Greg was diagnosed with aggressive stage 3 colon cancer. The cancer cells had not only attacked his colon but had also moved into his lymphatic system.

When Greg started his journey with his fiercest opponent, he became the ultimate cheerleader for anyone that God put in his path. He realized that God didn't intend for cancer to curse or harm him, but that God intended it for something good. Greg understood

God comforts us in all our troubles, so that we can comfort those in any trouble with the comfort we ourselves receive from God.

2 Corinthian 1:4

that it is during our times of deepest pains and weaknesses that we have the most to give.

Greg didn't see cancer as a curse. He saw it as an opportunity to share God with others. He began seeing people through a different lens.

In Greg's book, *Out of the Blue*, he shares with the reader his encounters with others. He allows you to see the joy that following Jesus brings.

"Cancer builds bridges and breaks down walls. You see suffering has an upside. It draws us to each other and God."

Greg is the forever cheerleader. Even after his passing, Greg continues to encourage others with his written word.

Greg Murtha made very accurate statements while dealing with cancer. One of my favorites is this: "Often, the place where we've suffered is where we have the most to give."

There are positives that evolve from a cancer diagnosis. People all over the world have taken their experiences and used them to help others. It may be something small that impacts a community, or it may be something big that changes the world.

In our small community, there have been several who have received a cancer diagnosis. Three years ago, a man and a woman were diagnosed with brain cancer the same week. GO STRONG became their slogan. T-shirts were made and over 600 sold. The money was donated to several causes. Still today, the shirts are worn throughout our small community. When anyone sees the words GO STRONG, it is a reminder that you can walk strongly with God no matter what type of mud you are walking through.

A child named Price in our community was diagnosed with brain cancer. His family has embraced the joy of being able to share monetary donations with St. Jude's Children's Hospital in Memphis. One of the ways they give is through the **Hunting for a Cure Youth Turkey Hunt**. Last year, they raised more than $150,000. Price's dad took Price on this hunt, and now he takes Price's friends. They also had community members buy a fruit tree and plant it in a large field. It is "Price's Orchard." Once the trees bear fruit, the fruit will be shared with others. Price's football number, #57, is still worn during different events to remember the powerful, influential young man who once wore the number on his chest. His jersey is also on display in the Ricebird fieldhouse for all players to remember him and his uplifting attitude toward life.

Price's quote that is still a quote throughout our community today is *"Either way, I will be okay."* Price may have only been 14, but he had wisdom beyond his years. He taught lessons to young and old during his time on this earth and even now after his passing.

One of the largest foundations is the **Susan G. Komen Race for a Cure** (www.komen.org) started by Nancy G. Brinker after the death of her sister, Susan G. Komen; this organization is a worldwide leader in the fight against breast cancer.

The **Lance Armstrong Foundation**, most commonly referred to as Livestrong.org, is another well-known cancer foundation. Cancer survivor Lance Armstrong founded this organization. The foundation's purpose is to provide education and support to individuals living with cancer, as well as to their loved ones and those charged with their care.

Another charity that provides funding for cancer research and support services for cancer patients and survivors is the **Vineman Cancer Charities Fund** (www.vineman.com). This fund was started to honor cancer survivor Barbara Recchia. Their largest fundraiser is "Barb's Race," an annual all-women's half ironman distance race held in Santa Barbara.

Jimmy Valvano is known for his quote, "Don't give up …. don't ever give up!" These words are on the home page of the **Jimmy V Victory Over Cancer** website (www.jimmyv.org). His foundation, which he formed months before his death, has raised millions of dollars for cancer research nationwide. Jimmy Valvano was a legendary basketball coach who was able to think beyond his life.

Molly MacDonald's breast cancer was a relatively mild case, but it did disrupt her life. She understands that there are many women who have more disruptions than she did. She began to wonder what happens when women can't work and have to take care of their families. Molly formed the **Pink Fund** (www.pinkfund.org) that provides financial support to help meet basic needs, decrease stress levels, and allow breast cancer patients to focus on healing while improving survivorship outcomes.

Jessica DeCristofaro is a stage 4 cancer survivor and the "Lymphoma Barbie" blogger. She has worked in the dermatology field for over five years, and skincare is her passion. Jessica wants cancer patients to still be able to feel beautiful even when going through intensive chemotherapy. She has created "Chemo Kits" (www.chemo-kits.com) that will help you get through chemo and boost your mood. Jessica also wrote the Cancer 101 book entitled *Talk Cancer to Me: My Guide to Kicking Cancer's Booty.*

The Little Rock 20th Century Club, a non-profit organization, began the **Hope Lodge** (www.hopeaway fromhome.org). This lodge provides a comfortable, convenient place to stay for cancer patients who are receiving treatment in Arkansas. The lodge offers meals, snacks, and fellowship. Transportation is also available for rides to area cancer facilities. Lodging is provided at no cost. Patients are chosen by social workers at the local cancer treatment centers. The club also started the **Angels of Hope Program** for high school juniors. This program promotes an attitude of Service Above Self. Each angel has to complete 25 hours of service. Twenty hours are earned through required activities at local hospitals with cancer treatment facilities and cancer-related events.

Brothers and sisters, think of what you were when you were called. Not many of you were wise by human standards; not many were influential; not many were of noble birth. But God chose the foolish things of the world to shame the wise; God chose the weak things of the world to shame the strong. God chose the lowly things of this world and the despised things—and the things that are not—to nullify the things that are, so that no one may boast before him.

1 Corinthians 1:26–29

BROKENNESS
OPENS THE
DOOR FOR US
TO DO FOR
OTHERS. WE
WOULD HAVE
NEVER OPENED
THE DOOR IF
WE HAD NOT
BEEN BROKEN.

13.
YOU ARE A CHAMPION

As Tom Burnett and his fellow passengers were devising a plan of action, Tom called his wife. The last words she heard him speak were, "We're going to do something," and they did. Tom and his fellow passengers rose from their seats and were the first to ever fight back against terrorism. Because of their bravery and plan of action, they saved thousands of lives.

Our purpose for writing the book *Game On* is also to save lives. We, like the passengers of Flight 93, are rising from our seats and making a plan of action. We aren't staying in the stands. We are joining you on the field. We are taking action and doing something that will help not only our local community but our global community as well.

Our passion is to help you make the touchdowns and be a champion.

CHAMPIONSHIPS

I can't promise you a victory, but I do know that with God you can have hope. Only God knows the plan for your life. All we ask of you is that you make these the best days you can. You make this disease worthwhile. Don't let cancer determine who you are. Take the situation you are in and glorify Him. People are watching, stay in faith, and move down the field toward the goal. Take note of the touchdowns along the journey and praise Him.

I loved the words that were spoken on the cheerleader video. I listened diligently and wrote down everything. I couldn't say it any better than they did:

> Championships aren't given, they are earned. You listen to their voice; you hear what they need. You watch the plays, and you know whether we are playing offense or defense. Your feet hit the floor, and you are ready to move. There is work to do. There is an easy way to the path of least resistance. The easy way out will always be there. Decide what you want to do. With each step comes the decision to take another. You are on your way. You are in a fight with an opponent you can't see, but you can feel him on your heels. Feel him breathing down your neck. That is your fear and doubt ready to shoot you out of the sky, but don't lose heart. They aren't easily defeated. It is a battle between your mind and the devil on your shoulders telling you this is just a game, a waste of time. Your opponents are stronger than you. Burn away your self-doubt with the fire burning beneath you. Remember what you are fighting for. Remember momentum is a cruel mistress. He is always searching for the weak place in your armor. The devil is looking for what you forgot to prepare for. As long as the devil is hiding in the details, the question is, Is that all you got? Are you sure? When you have prepared yourself for battle, it is time to go forward and face your enemy. Only now you take the fight into the open into hostile territory. Lion in a field of lions all hunting the elusive pray with the motivation that victory is the only thing in sight. So, play with the determination that you can run faster and play better.

205

Some people are cheerleaders even if they can't fit in their uniform.

Misti Coker

Sweat is a choice. Destiny waits for no man. When your time comes and a thousand voices are telling you you aren't ready for it, listen to the lone voice that says you are ready and you are prepared.

This is YOUR game. What will the score be? **Game On.**

TEAMMATES: PATIENT SURVEYS

*Let each of
you look not
only to his own
interests, but
also to the
interests of
others.*

Philippian 2:4

Cancer patients and family members share helpful tips for successful plays on the field.

PATIENT: KEITH

Cancer: Lung, stage 3a

Cancer Is ... the devil's tool to take us out, God's tool to build our faith.

Three Pieces of Advice:
* See a good naturalist and eat healthy. Take supplements, no more sugar.
* Get knowledgeable about your type of cancer.
* Pray and believe.

How Do You Stay Positive? Pray and believe. Speak and declare healing. Ignore negative outcome stories. Believe that your story will be a positive outcome.

Insurance Advice: Everyone should have a cancer insurance plan. See a good agent to look over your existing plans and policies and be sure you know everyone's coverage to make sure the survivor is taken care of.

How Do You Keep Healthy? Eat healthy fresh foods and supplements—d3 at night, b-100 for day. Eat protein.

Your Cancer Team: We were it—my husband and me.

Chemotherapy: Hair loss. Appetite change. Be careful of natural supplements that may prohibit chemo from working. Once again find out about everything you are doing—knowledge.

Explain Your Radiation Experience: Drains you! You feel worn out. Did not have any burning, but did have some indigestion, heartburn, and difficulty swallowing.

Any Other Information: A naturalist suggested that my husband soak in a warm tub of water three times weekly (up to his chin since his radiation was in his chest/esophageal) with one cup of sea salt and two cups of baking soda. Drain the tub then stand and shower off. The idea is to pull out the excess radiation so it doesn't just stay in the body to harm other organs. This helped with energy levels also. We felt this was very effective.

PATIENT: BRENT

Cancer: Lung/Liver

Cancer Is … scary, priority is to clear, eye opening, learning experience, tiring, draining, a time for God to show up and show out. Brings family closer together and life altering.

Three Pieces of Advice:
- No matter what, remember: God is bigger than any cancer.
- Stay positive.
- Be the germ police.

How Do You Stay Positive? With the help of your support group, such as family and friends, with lots of prayer.

Insurance Advice: Keep a notebook of all your bills and your EOBs. We had a supplemental cancer policy, and every month I turned in everything they required, and the next day I had a check in my account. I hope everyone I know has a cancer policy; it is well worth it.

How Do You Keep Healthy? I take B complex vitamins, drink protein shakes, Gatorade, and PowerAde, and eat lots of protein.

Your Cancer Team: My oncologist, Dr. Baltz, chemo nurses, nurses at doctor's office, Dr. Hord (PCP), and my surgeon, Dr. Burnett, are great health providers. My spouse, children, mom and dad, family and friends, plus other people in our small town who are going through the same experience have been wonderfully supportive.

Chemotherapy: The chemo nurses were very positive, knowledgeable, and caring. I could not taste food, my joints hurt, and my hands and feet swelled and tingled. I was very tired, had some nausea and vomiting, lost some hair, and gained weight. I had to take pain meds, steroids, anti-

DON'T BE TACKLED ON THE ONE YARD LINE. KEEP GOING AND MAKE THE TOUCHDOWN!

nausea meds, sleeping pills, magic mouthwash, B complex vitamins, and antibiotics.

Any Other Information: Do what the doctor tells you to do. Do not hesitate to let the doctor know any little changes that are happening. It is very important even if you think it might not matter, it does! Don't be afraid to ask questions.

PATIENT: JUDY

Cancer: Rectal Colon

Cancer Is … everywhere, every day, anyone.

Three Pieces of Advice:
- Pray more than you ever have.
- Believe in your doctors, nurses, and caregivers.
- Be thankful and grateful. There is always someone in the chemo lab or doctor's office who is sicker than you are.

How Do You Stay Positive? It can be difficult to stay positive when you don't feel good. You must have faith the size of a mustard seed; it can move mountains. Mountains are pretty big, so have BIG FAITH.

Insurance Advice: Visit with the social worker in your doctor's office. There are some grants for medicines. Some medicines can be very expensive. The social worker at my doctor's office got my pain patch paid for through a grant. If she had not, it would have cost me $1,700 a month. Being self-employed was a struggle. When I didn't work, I didn't have an income. There was a balance after insurance, so I would make monthly payments. I'm still paying, but getting them knocked out. Being sick is expensive, but I found that there are nice, patient people. There is help for those with insurance and those without.

How Do You Keep Healthy? I stay rested and try to stay away from germs. I wash my hands a lot and try to stay away from trips to the store.

Your Cancer Team: Daughters, husband, friends, support group, cancer friends. I wanted to be on every prayer list. There were people praying for me I didn't even know.

Chemotherapy: I was very sick during chemo. I suggest fluids, fluids, and more fluids (such as Ensure and Gatorade), but my treatment was in 2014; they have come a long way in a few short years. I ate Russell Stover lemon drops for the metal taste, and I also love phenergan for nausea.

Explain Your Radiation Experience: It sneaks up on you. You think it is going to be fine, and then boom, it hits you—no energy. I didn't have any burning—just weakness.

Any Other Information: You think it will never happen to you, but it does. In life, there are those bumps in the road, and I am sure I drove my family and friends crazy. I cried a lot and still do, but I cry because I am so grateful for great doctors, support groups, and church family, and I can't fathom not believing in the Big Doctor. I wrote everything down because something you say will be motivational to someone else who is going through cancer.

Postscript: Bigen hair color for chemo and radiation patients is chemical free. If your hair's turning gray—no more gray with this product.

Patient: Sarah

Cancer: Hodgkin's Lymphoma

Cancer Is … eye opening and life changing. Some are good changes and some are bad, but without question, it is life changing.

Three Pieces of Advice:
- Don't google anything. Find a doctor you trust and follow their advice. Ask them questions, but don't read information on the Internet.
- Make sure you have a good support system.
- You will hear all sorts of comments from people. Some are offensive, but try to remember that someone who has not gone through cancer can't understand and may not say the right things.

How Do You Stay Positive? Reading a daily devotional, finding quotes that made me mentally stronger, and again surrounding myself with a good support group.

Insurance Advice: Do not pay any bills until it shows on your EOB. Match your bills to your EOBs to make sure they have been turned in to your insurance company. Also find out what your maximum out-of-pocket is, and do not pay a penny over that amount. Get a cancer policy.

How Do You Keep Healthy? I decided if I felt bad I was going to eat how I wanted. I know that isn't good.

Your Cancer Team: My mom—my rock, my #1 fan. She was always there. My husband now, but my fiancé at the time of my diagnosis, was truly there for me.

Chemotherapy: I had four different chemos every other week, referred to as the ABCD. The red devil was part of that and was supposed to be the worst. About two days after chemo, I would feel like a big truck ran over me. My bones would ache so badly, and I would just cry. I literally wore out heating pads from lying on them so often. My overall chemo experience was good though because it killed the cancer, but it was the hardest four months of my life.

Explain Your Radiation Experience: I only had a few weeks of radiation. What radiation does to the body is unexplainable. You are more tired than you could have ever imagined. So rest your body; it needs it to get well.

Any Other Information: No one knows everything but God. If you have been given bad news, always stay positive and hopeful. A great fertility doctor told me that I would probably never have children

Cancer is a team sport. It doesn't just deal with one individual; it is about teammates working together and trusting each other to make the touchdowns.

Misti Coker

on my own, that there was less than a 10% chance. Within two years of being told that, I found out I was pregnant. Today I have two beautiful baby girls. Only God has a plan for you.

One thing my doctor said to me was this: *You are one of the lucky ones.* This was when I was first diagnosed and could not understand why on earth she would say that. Then I learned why. If you get a cancer diagnosis and you beat the cancer, you truly have a new outlook and understanding of what is really important, so you are one of the lucky ones.

PATIENT: SHERRY

Cancer: Breast 1991/stage 4 metastatic cancer of the internal mammary lymph node

Cancer Is ... a journey taken one day at a time.

Three Pieces of Advice:
- Attitude is everything.
- Out of all bad comes good.
- Fight back.

How Do You Stay Positive? I didn't let cancer dominate me emotionally or spiritually.

Insurance Advice: Seek out the insurance representative in your physician's office. I was fortunate I had taken out a cancer policy.

How Do You Keep Healthy? Listen to your body. There are wonderful nutritional cancer books out there. Find the foods that you can eat.

Your Cancer Team: Friends and family were there to comfort me, drive me to radiation, cook for me, and just help me get through. My doctors and staff at the Winthrop Rockefeller Cancer Institute, especially Dr. Makhoul and Dr. Klimburg, were wonderful.

Chemotherapy: So much has changed and improved since 1991. There are great medicines out there for everything—take them. My taste did change, and I couldn't eat anything with tomatoes.

Explain Your Radiation Experience: Fatigue! You can't explain the exhaustion you feel. Be patient; it will get better, but it may take several months. You will probably get some burning inside and out, but this will heal.

Any Other Information: I have survived cancer twice, in 1991 and 2006. In 2006, my diagnosis was grim—stage 4 metastatic cancer of the internal mammary lymph node—but I survived. I believe a positive attitude is everything, and out of all bad comes good. My thanks are to all of those who shared my illness with me. My friends and family were always there. My community was wonderful, sending cards, meals, praying, and much more. To God who has given me the gift of this day, I am grateful. *This is the day the Lord has made. We will rejoice and be glad in it.* Psalm 118:24

PATIENT: NANCY

Cancer: Hodgkin's Lymphoma (Hodgkin's Disease)

Cancer Is ... a change of life; you are more aware of what is happening with your body, and you wake every morning and thank God for another day of life.

Three Pieces of Advice:
- When people offer to help—LET THEM. They need to help as much as you need help.
- Never give up. God has a plan for you; you may not see it yet.
- Give even strangers a chance to help. They will be friends long after you are better.

How Do You Stay Positive? I never thought I would not make it. Even strangers told me I would survive. I also had support from my family and church.

Explain Your Radiation Experience: I went through nine weeks of radiation, four weeks from the bottom of my ribs to out the back of my head. They let me heal for four weeks and then went back for five more weeks from my ribs to my waist.

Any Other Information: There was a time when I couldn't eat due to the radiation burning my esophagus. I do have some long-term damage from scar tissue in my lungs, and I also have dry mouth.

PATIENT: SANDRA

Cancer: Breast

Three Pieces of Advice:
- Learn as much as you can about your kind of cancer.
- Keep very good notes about your doctor appointments, and keep a file of your tests.
- Stay positive. Trust God to deliver you through the treatments to good health. Let your friends and family help you fight cancer.

How Do You Stay Positive? I cling to God's promises to work all things for good in my life. I take comfort in every hug, kindness, and prayer I get from so many who have come to my aid.

Insurance Advice: Check out your exact coverage so you can understand all the bills that come in your mailbox.

How Do You Keep Healthy? I am studying nutrition books for cancer patients. I am in the process of developing a diet for myself. I have 40 pounds to lose to be at my ideal weight.

Your Cancer Team: Breast surgeon, oncologist, radiologist, and family.

Chemotherapy: I had four chemo treatments. I was very fatigued for about 10 days and nauseated after each treatment. I was short of breath some and had headaches and body aches. By the third week, I felt okay before my next treatment.

Any Other Information: Exercise when you feel well enough. Get plenty of rest. Think positive and be grateful.

PATIENT: KATHLEEN

Cancer: Ovarian, stage 3

Three Pieces of Advice:
- DON'T FREAK OUT! (That is what I told my husband.)
- Discuss all the treatment options with doctors and family and pick the best for you.
- Carry on your life as much as normal as you can.

How Do You Stay Positive? How do you not stay positive? I have a lot to live for: family and grand-kids who I want to watch grow up and enjoy.

Insurance Advice: Luckily, I have good insurance, but I do know if they don't want to pay something, go to your doctor or the company making the drug. Argue your case always.

How Do You Keep Healthy? I'm not good at that. I don't eat healthily. I eat as normally as I did before. I do avoid spicy foods.

Your Cancer Team: My main caregiver is Paul, my husband, but my family and especially my friends help also.

Chemotherapy: My treatment was very positive. I received 12 chemo treatments before my surgery (total hysterectomy and debulking). One month after surgery, I got a port and started back on treatments. My last chemo count was #73. Chemo was not bad on me; my main complaint is neuropathy in my feet and hands. The chemo was carboplatin, cisplatin, doxil (red devil), and topotecan. I had steroids and a B12 shot every treatment.

Explain Your Radiation Experience: I only have had radiation on my head where they radiated five small spots. Since then I have had clear scans. These treatments did make me a little brain tired. This is the best way to describe it.

Any Other Information: Use children's toothpastes and mouth rinse; adult products seem to burn the gums.

Use Cetaphil soap, lotion, etc.; this brand is easy on the skin during treatments. I used Nioxin or Bushey shampoo and conditioner to help hair growth.

Always remember what you are going through is temporary. When I got cancer, I said if a little girl like Asher Ray "Bit" can go through all of this, so can I. Four years later, she is still doing it, and two-fifths of a year, so am I. I just put Velcro strips on things that are slick and my fingertips slide on. (No, don't put the other side of the strip on you.) Hairspray cans, chiiron, works great!

Yes, I do drink alcohol—not that much, but it makes me feel like a normal person. Being normal is what I strive most to be like.

One of the most important things to do is find a support group. We didn't have one in our small town, so I started one. We are a group of around 30 women who have cancer or have had cancer. We meet once a month for dinner at a local restaurant. We also have a "GROUPME app" that we talk on every day. Someone is always there for you 24/7 every day of the week. We call ourselves the Chemosabes.

PATIENT: SHERRY

Cancer: Hodgkin's in 1982, returned three times; Breast in 2008

Cancer Is ... lonely and scary.

Three Pieces of Advice (plus one):
- Do not compare your cancer to someone else's. Trust your doctor.
- Look for the blessings and praise God for this time.
- Let people help you! They want to and you need them.
- It's okay to have a pity party on occasion; just don't make it a habit.

How Do You Stay Positive? Turn the bad into a blessing and stay connected to God; praise Him!

Insurance Advice: Keep your EOB and compare to bills when they come in. Get a good contact person who understands insurance and medical statements, and contact them when you have questions.

How Do You Keep Healthy? I wasn't too good in this area. I had a weird appetite. I drank protein drinks, ate yogurt, fruit, and protein powder, and I would use Half and Half to keep my weight up.

Your Cancer Team: I had a team with Hodgkin's named RAMS (Right Attitude Makes Sense). I was blessed with friends, family, and churches throughout the United States. I wrote to each one after every doctor's appointment and/or treatment and gave them an update. They took the time to pray; the least I could do was to keep them updated. That was before the social media we have today. With breast cancer, I was able to use Facebook to keep my team updated. I also kept a journal; just writing to my team members was a healthy outlet. I really encourage journaling and writing your feelings down.

Chemotherapy: In 1982, they didn't have the meds they have today. I was very sick the first week of every treatment. I was vomiting every two hours on the hour, so I tried a variety of nausea meds. Finally, at the end, I found a plan that made it better. I mainly drank water because of taste and sucked on lemon drops.

Explain Your Radiation Experience: The negative part of this was the everyday drive to Little Rock. I was pretty red and my skin was dry. They told me to use Aquaphor cream to restore the skin.

Any Other Information: Count your blessings, not your worries. Laugh, laugh, laugh, have fun. Play music, sing loud, and dance with your husband in the middle of the living room. Treasure each day and each new experience; smell the flowers. Exercise your mind body and spirit. If you are a woman with cancer, listen carefully. We have a tendency to take care of everyone else. It is time for you to take care of you. Take charge of your health.

PATIENT: MARY NINA

Cancer: Squamous Cell, started as anal, then moved to thigh and shoulder, and is now in two lymph nodes in my left groin area.

Cancer Is ... not a journey as most people say. I have learned a lot about myself during my fight, and I have also learned it is all small stuff. The only things that really matter are God and family. I feel more at peace than I ever have in my life. How crazy is that? It took cancer to slow me down and make me realize what is important. Through this whole time, I have said, "Treatment is just some shit I have to go through to get well—and I will get well!"

Three Pieces of Advice:
- It isn't a death sentence. Explore all of your options, then fight like hell.
- Take it one day at a time.
- Let people help you with meals, laundry, cleaning house, and driving to appointments. Whatever it is, accept the help and move on. I admit it was hard at first, but it makes it so much easier for you to focus on your health and getting better.

How Do You Stay Positive? I get up every day thankful for another day. I have laughed at myself, thinking maybe I am in denial about having cancer because I have not let it get me down mentally. I do what I feel like physically, but have been able to stay very positive. I would not have made it through this without my faith, my totally amazing husband, and my family and friends. I have a wonderful support system.

Insurance Advice: My primary insurance has paid almost everything, so I really don't have any advice. I do have a cancer policy, and I have to send in the EOB sheets from my primary insurance and bills to get reimbursed. Stay on top of this, or you will have to copy months' worth of papers at a time. If you do it monthly, it is not so overwhelming, and you will get a reimbursement check more frequently.

How Do You Keep Healthy? I have done terribly in this area. I have only been nauseated a few times and have been so glad. Since I haven't really been sick, I eat whatever I want. And I have gained a lot of weight. Try to make sensible choices about food and stay hydrated. It really will make you feel better. I drank so much G2 PowerAde Zero during my first round of chemo that I have a hard time drinking it now. Smart water is good too. Exercise if you feel like it. I hear it makes you feel better. I haven't really tried it though.

Your Cancer Team: All my doctors, oncologist, radiation oncologist, surgeons, wound care center, and my family have been wonderful.

Chemotherapy: My first round of chemo I received 5 FU five days a week for 10 weeks. Food tasted weird, but not too bad. And that ended after a few weeks. Also, I did not have a port the first round. Get one. Getting stuck every other day was awful. After about five weeks into my treatments, so many of my veins had blown that I had to get a PICC line to finish. That was a godsend. I would not have been able to finish without it. Second time around I got a port. I love it and will not get it removed until I am absolutely 100% positive I will not have to have any more chemo. When I was taking Taxol and carbo, everything tasted like metal. Lemonheads helped. It only lasted a couple of months. My taste buds weren't back to normal, but at least there was no more metal taste. If you do not already take an antidepressant, ask for a prescription. It helps. Zofran helps with nausea. Ativan (Lorazepam) helps with sleep. I take it every night. As of September 15, 2016, I have had 92 chemo treatments. These began March 10, 2015, and I will continue to get it for the rest of my life if that is what it takes. The chemos I have taken are as follows: 5 FU–50 treatments; Pacitaxol and Carboplatin–22 treatments; Navelbine–22 treatments and counting.

Explain Your Radiation Experience: Radiation was not too bad other than the fatigue. That is unlike anything I have ever been through. I was lucky and didn't really burn the first time, just some irritation. Radiation beam was to my abdominal area, but target spot was my anal area. I was thrown into menopause, but that was fine with me. Radiation to my left leg causes no side effect. The radiation to my left shoulder left a big rectangle burn on my back. It had to be treated for about two weeks and then it was gone. I do still have pain in my shoulder that my doctors think is inflammation from the radiation. I started radiation in April of 2015 and as of September 15, 2016, I have had 52 radiation treatments—all spots combined.

Any Other Information: It is now August 2017 and my tumor has grown. My chemo concoction that MD Anderson created has not worked. Back to the drawing board. Next week I will begin a clinical trial at MD Anderson. I will travel back and forth from Arkansas to Texas hoping that this will be the answer. Never give up—try everything. There is something out there that will work for you.

PATIENT: AMY

Cancer: Chronic Myelogenous Leukemia

Cancer Is ... something I will live with for the rest of my life. CML currently has no cure. I am blessed to have a cancer that is very treatable. Cancer for most patients is devastating and terminal; however, I am continually amazed at those who keep a positive attitude in spite of their diagnosis.

Three Pieces of Advice:
- Wait; don't freak out. Take it all in and gather information.
- It is ok to be tired; take advantage of the down time.
- Work through the stages even though you think they will never apply to you.

How Do You Stay Positive? Faith and believing in God, continuing to work and go about my daily living, focusing on others instead of self, meditation, journaling, and reading my Bible worked for me.

Insurance Advice: Fortunately, I had taken out a cancer policy at work while forgetting that I was still paying for a portable cancer policy from another employer. This is yet another part of God's perfect timing.

How Do You Keep Healthy? Lol! I take my meds as directed, try to eat healthier, cleaner foods, not really much change.

Your Cancer Team: My oncologist and his caring staff, my boss and PCP, my precious family and friends, church family, and fantastic coworkers.

Chemotherapy: Oral chemo twice daily. Timing issues two hours before and one hour after eating. It makes me turn beet red.

Any Other Information: CML is much different than other cancers. It is difficult to look fine but to have something wrong with you that causes horrible fatigue. The Sunday before I was diagnosed,

I was reading in our episcopal devotional book (February 8) and this is what it said:

> We are all weary at times, physically, spiritually, and emotionally. The drudgery, stress, and challenges of life can wear us down. What are the monsters that approach you in the mist when you are very weary? Unlike us, God does not grow tired or faint. What good news.

It is interesting to see God's plan at work through many things that I have read and experienced. He has perfect timing. I pray for all of those with cancer, but find the way I get through it is to not think about it. I must think about something other than cancer.

Patient: Spouse of Cancer Patient

Cancer: Breast

Cancer Is ... a pause button. Cancer stops your life and demands your full attention. It's not logical, there's no reasoning with it, and you are at its mercy.

Three Pieces of Advice:
- How everyone mentally approaches the diagnosis will determine how treatment goes. Don't get stuck asking why or how did this happen. It happened; just focus on beating it (easier said than done).
- People are going to start treating you differently, and most people don't know how to react. Be prepared to answer lots of the same (sometimes stupid) questions over and over.

- The hardest part of cancer is after you've beaten it. Picking up where you left off is going to be difficult. Everyone else's lives continued on as normal while you've been fighting this battle to keep living. You'll realize people take a lot of things for granted, and it'll make you angry. Every hiccup, cough, or sneeze will be alarming. You've got a new friend that gets to tag along with your 2, 5, 10, 20 year plans. What you want to be when you grow up has a bit more urgency to it.

How Do You Stay Positive? I stayed positive because Jessica was. We all realized there wasn't anything else to do besides put our heads down and get through treatment.

Insurance Advice: Have good insurance. They will nickel and dime you for every last bit. Even with great insurance, make sure you have money saved up for all the other non-medical costs. You're going to be taking a lot of time off, spending money on hospital meals and fast food. There's nothing like being fed through the health system to make you understand how messed up it is. Every day you'll see and experience things inside hospitals and with other patients that were beyond your comprehension.

How Do You Keep Healthy? It didn't seem like Jessica had much of a choice of what she wanted to eat. Most of the time she was too sick to eat. Whenever she was hungry, we'd feed her whatever she could keep down. Diets during chemo are like war. All the best laid plans fly right out the window as soon as the battle starts.

Your Cancer Team: Parents and close friends. Lots of people will reach out who you haven't talked to in a long time and will try and help out.

Chemotherapy: I took a seemingly healthy person into the hospital, and 30 minutes later she was a zombie who looked like she was recovering from a two-month vodka bender. Other than that, it was fine.

Any Other Information: Cancer makes your whole life stop. Nothing else matters anymore. Your job, your hobbies, your plans all go out the window and you focus on nothing else but breathing the cancer. This is true for the patient and their support system.

Treatment is a blur. You'll learn the ins and outs of the hospital and thank God every day that you're lucky to have insurance, family, and a good support system. Seeing people go through treatment without it is heartbreaking.

After treatment is over, the healing really begins. All your doctors who were all up in your business now only want to see you twice a year, and you need to wait two weeks if something weird is happening before scheduling an appointment.

You'll be recovering physically for at least a year and mentally even longer. You probably won't be able to think as quickly or remember things as easily.

PATIENT: JESSICA

Cancer: Breast Cancer-Infiltrating Ductal Carcinoma, stage 2B, ER+, PR+, Her2Nu-)

Cancer Is ... evil, uprooting, confusing, scary, life changing.

Three Pieces of Advice:
- Get a second opinion regarding your treatment plan.
- Be sure you LIKE your doctor(s). They need to be good at what they do, but also kind, understanding, and approachable, and YOU must ultimately be comfortable with them.
- Surround yourself with family and friends. It is impossible to do this alone.

How Do You Stay Positive? Luckily, my cancer was not life-threatening (at least, as non-life threatening as cancer can be). So that is something I held onto. I knew if I could get through the treatments and surgery, that there was light at the end of that tunnel and I would be through. I don't know that there's a science to staying positive. For me, positivity was the only thing that got me through each day—so it wasn't really a choice. I could be positive and get through it, or not and suffer more. Family and friends also helped me to stay positive. The biggest thing is to not let the cancer consume or define you. If you accept cancer as being a part of your life, but not the defining part, it is much easier to stay positive.

Insurance Advice: Whew, insurance can be a mess. And it's so hard to understand. Many of us (including myself) who are intelligent people still find deciphering insurance policies and healthcare forms to be incredibly confusing and difficult. Get with someone at your doctor's office who can help you increase your "health literacy." Some insurance companies will assign you a case officer (mine did!). Ask them as many questions as you need to. That is what they're there for if you need to call someone at your insurance company. Understand what your policy covers and what it doesn't, what your deductible is and how much you'll have to pay out of pocket before insurance covers things, etc. Also, cross check your "explanation of benefits" from your insurance company with bills from your doctor/hospital. If they don't match, tell someone. Oftentimes, there's an error, and you don't actually owe that much. SAVE EVERYTHING medical-related (receipts, bills, explanations of benefits, etc.). You may need it in the future to file an appeal. Ask your doctor/hospital about payment plans if there is a large bill you can't pay right away. Most will do that without interest.

How Do You Keep Healthy? It was hard. During chemo, I became repulsed by most vegetables, and it was hard to stomach anything but carbs (which is not great, especially for cancer patients). During radiation, I just wasn't hungry. Every single time you crave, or get even close to craving a vegetable or fruit, EAT IT. I tried to find healthy alternatives to wheat I could eat. for example, I ate a lot of bread so I tried to eat whole grain instead of white. I cut out processed sugars and foods as much as I could. I tried to eat fresh. For produce I purchased organic, or when that became too expensive, I cleaned my fruits and veggies with a vinegar solution. I also tried to go vegan for a couple of weeks, and I felt great, but it became too hard to continue once treatment started. I was too tired to food prep and cook. I really enjoyed the book *Crazy Sexy Diet* by Kris Carr. She has been living with an incurable cancer for seven years after changing her diet. When diagnosed she was given seven months to live.

Your Cancer Team: My mom and my dad were my biggest supporters. I lived with them throughout the whole process and could not have gotten through it without them. My boyfriend was living in Kansas City at the time, which was very hard. But he supported me as best he could from there and visited often. My brother was living in Fayetteville but was also very supportive. He engaged his entire church/faith community to be constantly praying for me and for my healing, which was pretty amazing. My own church was also a great support. I found comfort and healing through my bible study groups, through church services, and through Sunday school. Having that community was wonderful. I was an outlier in that I did not find support groups to be helpful. For me personally, I would reach out to friends who had been through breast cancer, rather than a support group. However, I know they are helpful for a lot of people and suggest everyone at least try one.

Chemotherapy: Chemo was hard. My doctor did not prescribe a strong enough anti-nausea medication after my first round, so that was miserable. Once I got the right medication to help me deal with the symptoms, it was okay. I didn't experience a lot of nausea, which was great. But I would always feel fatigued, which made doing anything at all pretty difficult. My taste changed a bit, but mostly my cravings changed. I couldn't really stomach vegetables, and I began to HATE the taste of carrots (still do, actually), which I loved before. After three of my chemos I had to receive a shot to build my immune system back up, which gave me horrible joint pains that required narcotics to get through. The buildup of narcotics caused me to be extremely constipated for weeks, which was very uncomfortable. For all my medications, I had to test my limits and figure out what worked best for me so I could alleviate chemo symptoms but also not experience too many negative medication side effects.

Chemo brain is a thing, not just during chemo, but also after. In fact, I still deal with it. I was, and am, very forgetful, and I have a bad short-term memory. I even find it hard to recall long-term memories sometimes. My train of thought is also slower, which affects my speech.

Explain Your Radiation Experience: Radiation was, in some ways, harder than chemo. Doctors can't explain why, but most patients feel incredibly fatigued throughout radiation. For me, I was more fatigued during radiation than I was during chemo. It was hard. I didn't feel like doing anything. I wasn't hungry, and I was so tired. My skin was not really affected until my final two weeks. I used Aquaphor to calm the irritation, which helped, but it also put oily stains on my clothes that never washed out— so don't wear anything you don't mind messing up when you put that on. I have heard that second skin is also good but didn't use that. It took about two to three weeks after my final radiation treatment before my skin lesions healed.

Any Other Information: Before your surgery, get in touch with someone who has had that exact surgery so you can know what to anticipate. Your doctor will tell you, to some extent, but another patient will be able to give you tips and tricks for feeling good and getting around post-surgery that most doctors don't. I found it to be very helpful and was able to prepare a lot of things that I wouldn't have otherwise, like special shirts, special pillows, etc.

Ask your doctors every single question you think of, even if it sounds stupid or redundant. Learn everything about your illness and its treatment yourself by asking these questions so you can be informed. I found it hard to remember much of anything, so I wrote everything down, which was very helpful.

Don't be afraid to ask for help. It's not a sign of weakness. You have CANCER. You are being injected or radiated with POISON. You ARE weak. Let other people help you, and lean on them for physical and emotional support.

Be strong, be positive, pray often.

Questions for Your Doctors

General Questions for Your Oncologist
- Have you ever treated this type of cancer before?
- How successful were you?
- What medical facilities do you use?
- What insurance does your facility take?
- Discuss any issues you may be having—pain, problems.
- Discuss past health.

Treatment Questions for Your Oncologist
- What is your game plan for me?
- What treatment works best with my type of cancer?
- How many treatments will I have? (Ask for time-frame)
- Where will I have the treatment (outpatient or hospital)?
- What are the side effects?
- What risks are involved?
- Can this cancer spread?
- What is the expected outcome?
- What do I need to do to stay healthy during the treatment process?

- Do the treatments affect fertility or cause sexual issues?
- What treatment would you choose for your loved one?
- Can I work during treatment?
- What are the side effects of any medications?

QUESTIONS FOR YOUR SURGEON

- What experience do you have performing this surgery?
- What is your success rate with this type of surgery?
- How exactly is this operation performed?
- What are the risks, benefits, and possible complications?
- What hospital will the surgery take place?
- Should I stop taking certain medications?
- Are there any medications I will be taking after?
- Is there any special preparation before the test I need to do?
- Do I have any diet restrictions before, during, or after?
- How long is the recovery period? (In hospital stay or outpatient).
- What is the cost of the surgery, and what type of insurance do you take?
- How can I contact you if I have more questions?

ASK, ASK, ASK. Every question is important. Grab a notebook, write down all of your questions, and then ask at your appointment. You have to be your own advocate. If you feel uncomfortable asking questions, take someone with you who can.

GLOSSARY

acute: a rapidly developing condition. An acute medical condition comes on quickly and often causes severe symptoms but lasts only a short time.

allogeneic transplantation: a procedure where cells, tissue, or organs are transplanted to a person from a compatible donor.

alternative therapy: any healing practices that are not part of mainstream medicine—that means any practice that is not widely taught in medical schools or frequently used by doctors or in hospitals. Alternative medicine is often used *instead of* conventional medical techniques.

anemia: a condition in which the body has a low number of red blood cells.

anesthesia: the use of medicine to prevent the feeling of pain or sensation during surgery or other procedures that might be painful.

anesthesiologist: a physician who specializes in anesthesiology, the administering of anesthesia.

benign: not malignant, not harmful, non cancerous.

bilateral: found on both sides of the body; when referring to cancer, it means cancer found in paired organs (for example, in both kidneys).

biopsy: the removal of a sample of tissue from the body for further examination. A biopsy gives doctors a closer look at what's going on inside to help make a diagnosis and choose the right treatment.

blood: fluid that circulates within the human system.

blood banking: blood banks collect and store blood that healthy people donate. The bank keeps blood ready in case someone needs it because of an accident or surgery.

blood plasma: a yellowish liquid that carries nutrients, hormones, and proteins throughout the body.

bone marrow: a thick, spongy liquid inside the bones. Bone marrow makes all kinds of blood cells: red blood cells that carry oxygen, white blood cells that fight infections, and platelets that help blood clot.

bone marrow transplant (BMT): a procedure that involves replacing unhealthy bone marrow with healthy bone marrow cells from a donor.

cancer: when abnormal cells grow, divide, and spread very fast.

cancer care center: a center that offers patients everything they need in one place. There are many all over the United States. Their purpose is to provide cancer prevention, diagnosis, and treatment.

complete blood count (CBC): a common blood test that evaluates the three major types of cells in the blood: red blood cells, white blood cells, and platelets.

cells: the basic components or "building blocks" of the human body.

chemotherapy: chemicals that have specific toxic effect upon the disease.

chronic: an illness that someone has for a long time or one that goes away and keeps coming back.

Diabetes and juvenile rheumatoid arthritis, for example, are chronic illnesses.

CT: an x-ray image obtained with a cat scanner.

dietician/nutritionist: a person who is an expert in nutrition or dietetics.

disability (short term/long term): the state or condition of being disabled, lack of adequate power, strength, or physical or mental ability.

dysplasia: abnormal changes in the structure or organization of a group of cells.

edema: swelling in areas such as the feet and legs and the area around the eyes that is caused by excess fluid buildup in the tissues.

fatigue: weariness from bodily or mental exertion.

FMLA: family medical leave act, helps with job security. www.employment.findlaw.com/family-medical-leave/what-is-fmla-faq-on-federal-leave-law.html.

follow up: checkup after initial procedure.

genetics: the study of the way physical traits and characteristics get passed down from one generation to the next. This is also called **heredity**. Genetics includes the study of genes, which have a special code called DNA that determines what you will look like and whether you are likely to have certain illnesses.

grade: a grade for cancer that indicates how aggressive it is. The lower the grade, the less aggressive the cancer and the greater the chance for a cure. The higher the grade, the more aggressive the cancer and the harder it may be to cure.

hematology: the study of the nature, function, and diseases of the blood and of blood-forming organs

hemoglobin: a substance in red blood cells that carries oxygen through the blood to different parts of the body.

home health care services: wide range of healthcare services that can be given in your home due to an illness or injury, less expensive and more convenient.

hospice: a special type of care for people who are in the last phase of an illness. This type of care can be either inpatient or outpatient.

imaging scans: techniques that include x-rays, CT scans, MRI. These tools let your doctor see inside your body to get a picture of your bones, organs, muscles, tendons, nerves, and cartilage. This is the way the doctor sees any abnormalities.

immunotherapy: using the body's immune system to fight cancer.

incisional biopsy: a procedure in which the doctor opens the skin to remove a sample of suspicious tissue for purposes of diagnosis.

internal radiation: radiation therapy that usually requires a stay in the hospital for several days for careful monitoring. The radioactive material may be placed in small tubes that are implanted into the cancerous tumor or a body cavity, or swallowed or injected into the bloodstream.

inpatient: a patient who stays in a hospital while under treatment.

insurance: gives you protection and helps pay medical bills.

IV: a thin bendable tube that slides into one of the veins. It carries fluid, medicine, or blood to the body.

job security: probability that an individual will keep his or her job, FMLA.

laboratory tests: medical devices that are intended for use on samples of blood, urine, or other tissues or substances taken from the body to help with diagnose of disease or other conditions.

living will: written statement detailing a person's desires regarding their medical treatment in circumstances in which they are no longer able to express informed consent, especially an advance directive.

locally invasive: a tumor that can spread to the tissues surrounding it.

lumbar puncture: a procedure in which a small amount of fluid surrounding the brain and spinal cord (the cerebrospinal fluid) is removed and examined. See also *spinal tap*.

lumpectomy: a breast cancer procedure that involves removing a part of the breast containing a tumor known or suspected to be cancerous.

lymph: a clear, watery fluid containing protein molecules, salts, glucose, urea, and other substances that flows through its own vessels branching throughout the body. Lymph contains white blood cells, which are the germ fighters of the immune system.

lymph nodes: lymph nodes—little round or bean-shaped bumps that can't be felt unless they become swollen—are like filters that remove germs. They contain lymphocytes, white blood cells that fight infection.

lymph vessels: vein-like structures that help carry lymph (a clear, watery fluid containing protein molecules, salts, glucose, urea, and other substances) throughout the body.

lymphangiogram (LAG): a medical test that uses injection of a dye and x-rays to examine the lymphatic system.

lymphatic system: the network of tissues and organs that carry lymph (a clear, watery fluid containing protein molecules, salts, glucose, urea, and other substances) throughout the body.

lymphocyte: a type of white blood cell found in lymph nodes. Lymphocytes make antibodies, special proteins that fight off germs and stop infections from spreading by trapping disease-causing germs and destroying them.

Medicaid: funded by the government for low-income and needy people to help pay payments. www.ssa.gov/disabilityresearch/wi/medicaid.htm

Medicare: federal health insurance program for people who are 65 or older and certain younger people with disabilities. www.medicare.gov/sign-up-change-plans/decide-how-to-get-medicare/whats-medicare/what-is-medicare.html

MRI (Magnetic Resonance Imaging): a scan that uses a strong magnetic field and radio waves to create detailed images of the organs and tissues of the body. It is a tubular shaped structure.

malignant: another word for cancerous.

mammogram: a special kind of x-ray of the breast that helps doctors see what's going on inside.

medical history: information about a person's past health, their family's health, and other issues. All doctors want to know the ifs, ands, and buts of you.

metastasis: the spread of disease (in this case, cancer) from the original site to other parts of the body.

NPS (nurse practitioner) or APNS (advanced practice nurse): nurse who has completed an accredited educational program with a master's degree in nursing.

occupational therapist (OT): health professional trained to help people do the things they want and need to do. OTs intervene when a patient has had some sort of injury or disability. They set goals to help the patient perform daily activities.

oncologist: a doctor who is trained in the area of cancer.

outpatient: receiving treatment without being admitted to a hospital.

physician assistant (PA): Works under the supervision of a doctor and can prescribe medication.

pathologist: a scientist who studies the causes and effects of diseases, especially one who examines laboratory samples of body tissue for diagnostic or forensic purposes. The person who looks at the biopsy and determines whether it is cancer or benign. They identify the disease and its conditions.

PET: a scan that allows your doctor to check for any disease in your body. The scan uses a special dye that has radioactive tracers. These tracers are injected into a vein in your arm. Your organs and tissue then absorb the tracer.

physical therapist (PT): highly educated, licensed healthcare professional who can help patients reduce pain and improve mobility. PTs help to get your body going again without surgery or medicine.

platelets: tiny blood cells that circulate in your blood and help your body form clots to stop bleeding. A normal platelet count ranges from 150,000 to 450,000 per microliter of blood. Doctors get this count from a complete blood count (CBC).

port: long narrow soft plastic tube that is inserted into a vein to give medication. It is placed completely under your skin in your arm or chest. It is a lifesaver if you have to have many rounds of chemotherapy.

primary site: in this case, the organ or area in the body where cancer begins. Type of cancer is always identified by its primary site, even it metastasizes or spreads. For instance, if cancer begins in the liver but spreads to other organs, it is still classified as liver cancer.

prognosis: an estimate of how well a person's treatment is working and how likely or unlikely it is that the cancer will come back.

premiums (insurance): amount of money that an individual or business must pay for an insurance policy.

primary care physician (PCP): the doctor you contact when you are sick. He or she will then send you to specialists if needed.

protocol: a method or plan; in this case, the medications and treatments a patient will receive to help fight cancer.

psychiatrist, psychologist, psychotherapist: those trained to help with mental health issues, such as depression.

radiation: high-energy particles or waves, such as x-rays, gamma rays, electron beams, or protons, to destroy or damage cancer cells. Radiation can be used alone or with surgery and/or chemotherapy.

radiation oncologist: a specialist physician who uses radiation in the treatment of cancer.

recurrence: is the name giving if you have been cleared of cancer and then the cancer returns.

red blood cell count: a blood test where your doctor can find out your RBC counts. Your red blood cells carry oxygen to your blood.

regimen: a treatment plan or system. For cancer treatment, a regimen can include things like diet and exercise.

relapse: the reappearance of cancer after it has been treated.

remission: when cancer symptoms disappear or are significantly reduced.

RN (registered nurse): a nurse who is skilled to provide the best care to the patient and the family.

screenings and exams: tests that look for diseases before you have symptoms. Screenings and exams can help with early diagnosis.

side effect: an undesirable effect of a drug or medical treatment. Can be a number of things, such as fatigue, loss of appetite, weight gain, weight loss, headaches, nausea, pain, skin reactions.

social worker: a psychology-related field. A social worker is present to help families, individuals, and groups of people to cope with problems they are facing to improve their lives.

staging: a way to categorize patients according to how extensive the disease is at the time of diagnosis.

stem cells: primitive (early) cells found primarily in the bone marrow that are capable of developing into the three types of mature blood cells present in blood: red blood cells, white blood cells, and platelets.

stem cell transplant: a procedure that involves intro-ducing stem cells (cells found primarily in the bone marrow from which all types of blood cells develop) into the body in the hopes that the new cells will rebuild the immune system.

stop loss (insurance): insurance feature that protects patients from paying large claims. When the patient pays a certain amount out of pocket deter-mined by the insurance company, the patient doesn't have to pay anymore out of pocket.

surgeon: a medical practitioner qualified to practice surgery.

treatment plan: a road map the patient will follow on his or her journey through treatment.

trial: research studies that explore whether a medical strategy, treatment, or device is safe and effective for humans. These studies also may show which medical approaches work best for certain illnesses or groups of people.

tumor: abnormal body cells grouped together in a mass or lump. Tumors are classified as benign (not cancerous) or malignant (cancerous).

ultrasound: (also known as a sonogram) uses high fre-quency sound waves that give an internal view of your organs.

white blood cell count: the quantity of white blood cells in your blood. White blood cells help fight infections by attacking bacteria, viruses, and germs that invade the body. An increase in this count can indicate infection.

x-ray: a safe procedure that uses radiation to take pic-tures of internal areas of the body. They're done by an x-ray technician in the radiology department of a hospital, a freestanding radiology center, or a healthcare provider's office.

All definitions have been assembled from various online resources, including these:

- *www.thefreedictionary.com*
- *www.medical-dictionary.com*
- *www.kidshealth.org*
- *www.cancer.org*

Special Thanks

Special thanks to those listed below for sharing their stories, ideas, and expertise.

Dodd McCollum—United States Air Force

Kerry Seeman—KD Shack, Massage Therapist

Chemosabe Sisters—Cancer Women's Support Group

Nancy Duke—Cancer Survivor, designer of GAME ON Diagram

Amanda Norcross—Psychotherapist, LPC, MA in Psychology, MA in English

Nancy Harris Buckley—University of Arkansas Instructor, Dale Bumpers College of Agriculture, Food, and Life Sciences

Kelsie Konecny—Masters of Business Administration, Konecny Insurance Services CFO

Amelia Elam—Director, Policy and Education, Outreach Services at AFMC

Jennifer Sullivan—Trainer, Owner of True Fitness Gym

Marian Dickson Ruffin—RN, GriefShare Leader, Owner Turpin Funeral Home

Joan Gallagher—Author, *Hope Markers*, Speaker (www.joangallagher.net)

Vickie Henderson—OBGYN, Author, Speaker (www.myupsiderightlife.com)

Sherry Tuminello—Cancer Survivor, Librarian

Dr. John Sullivan—Cancer Patient, Bachelor of Divinity, Master of Divinity, Doctor of Ministry Degrees from Southwestern Baptist Theological Seminary

JB Grimes—Cancer Survivor, BSE, MSE, Coaching: Louisiana Monroe, Delta State, Missouri, Arkansas Razorbacks, Virginia Tech, Mississippi State, Arkansas State, Auburn, UCONN- Offensive Line Specialty Coach

Martha Ellen Talbot—Cancer Survivor, Fundraiser Expert, Owner of Marlsgate Plantation (www.marlsgate.com)

Jackie Coker Hill—MS Human Resources, Bristol Myers Squibb Executive Territory Sales Manager, Psychiatric Research Institute UAMS, Outreach Specialist at AFMC, Rodan and Fields Independent Skincare Consultant

Also a huge thank you to the many cancer patients, family members, friends, nurses, and doctors who took the time to sit down with me and share their stories.

Giving Back

A nudge, as I call it, is when the Lord prompts you to act upon a decision that is placed in your heart. Months ago, when I was in the beginning stages of Personal Pep Rally, I reached out to a family friend, Martha Ellen Talbot. Martha Ellen and I grew up in the Presbyterian church in Stuttgart, and her little sister and I were inseparable growing up. Her family was my second family as a child.

Martha Ellen left Stuttgart and made her home in Little Rock where she is involved in many fundraising and charity campaigns. One of her passions is being a member and officer of the 20th Century Club which funds the non-profit cancer patient lodge "Hope Away from Home."

Since some of the world's best cancer treatment facilities are located in Central Arkansas, many patients find their way to Little Rock. Finding a place to stay is a worry that cancer patients don't need on top of the other physical and emotional driving unknowns of cancer. This facility bridges a gap by providing a home away from home at no charge, healthy meals and snacks, plus a community of support.

As I sat and visited with Martha Ellen, I could feel her passion for people, and her want to give to others. As I asked her questions about the lodge and cancer, she briefly stopped and said, "You know I had breast cancer five years ago." I had no idea about her cancer battle. When people can genuinely put themselves in someone else's shoes, desire will yearn inside of them to do everything they can to be of assistance to others.

Last year Martha Ellen was co-chairman of the Hope Ball, and she is co-chairman again this year. The Hope Ball is an annual gala event hosted by the 20th Century Club to raise funding for the continued operation of the 20th Century Club's Hope Lodge. The annual event raises over $300,000 to sustain the expenses of the lodge.

I am grateful for the day the Lord nudged me to call Martha Ellen. She has given me words of wisdom to begin this journey of charitable work in creating Personal Pep Rally. Martha Ellen and I continue to meet once a month to keep me on track with developing ideas to motivate, encourage, and educate cancer patients and their families.

It is through our adversities that we gain desire in giving back to others. Martha Ellen is an example of just that.

Martha Ellen and her husband, Beau Talbot, own and operate Marlsgate Plantation located in Scott Arkansas.

Personal Pep Rally

Personal Pep Rally is a non-profit organization created to help cancer patients. *Game On* is part of the mission work done by this 501c3. More information can be found on their Facebook and Instagram pages and their website: personalpeprally.org.

Personal Pep Rally
Board of Directors

Misti Coker—BSE University of Arkansas, MSE Harding (Masters in Reading), Teacher, Life Coach (AACC), Author, Trainer for Process Communication

Jennifer Smith—ASU Finance Degree, Financial Advisor Edward Jones

Lana Flowers Roth—ASU Finance Degree, Juris Doctorate in Law University of Arkansas, General Counsel Producers Rice Mill

Natalie Wilks—Speech-Language Pathologist Masters, Rodan and Fields RFX Circle Achiever

Marlo Lock—UAMS RN Degree, Owner of All About You Salon & Aesthetics

Megan Ables—ASU Journalism Degree, MSE, Arkansas Teacher of the Year 2016, State Department of Education

Jenna Sexton—Sales and Marketing Assistant Producers Rice Mill

About the Authors

Jay and Misti Coker both grew up in a rural delta area of Arkansas. Stuttgart, Arkansas, the rice and duck capital of the world, has been their home for more than 50 years. They both attended and graduated from the University of Arkansas at Fayetteville. Jay has a BS in agriculture business, and Misti has a BS in education. Misti has received her Master's degree from Harding University in reading.

After college, Misti and Jay moved back to Stuttgart and began working in their areas of expertise. Misti taught school for 23 years. She taught second grade, first-grade reading, and seventh grade English, and later was Literacy Director for the Stuttgart School District. It was during this time that she also was trained in the Process Communication Model. It was her teaching experience and training that helped her raise test scores for the subpopulation that was underprivileged. She and her co-worker, Megan Ables, created the workshop "Teaching Secondary Is Elementary" that they shared with numerous improvement companies. She has since become an author, writing the children's book *A Little Bit of Hope* in honor of Asher Ray who battled cancer for five years. She also contributed a story about her daughter entitled "Fix It." This story is part of the book *I Heart Mom* by

Relevant Pages Press. Misti's goal is to help all cancer patients by motivating and encouraging them through her websites Personal Pep Rally (personalpeprally.org) and Pass on Joy (passonjoy.com).

Once Jay moved back to Stuttgart, he began his career in agriculture. He worked as a farm manager for a local farmer and then joined on with Southern Farmers Association as a field rep. Jay then became a rice consultant for Dunklin Farms. After several years, he branched out and gradually added to his acreage. Jay now farms over 6,000 acres of rice, beans, and corn. Jay is involved in many aspects of the farming community besides being in the field. He is co-owner of Dry Lake Hunting Service, which hunts over 300 hunters a season. He is chairman of the Arkansas Rice Research and Promotion Board, chairman of Producers Rice Mill Board, chairman of the Stuttgart Parks and Recreation Board, trustee of the Museum of the Arkansas Grand Prairie, and a member of the PCCUA at Stuttgart Foundation.

Jay and Misti are both active in their church, First United Methodist Church Stuttgart. Misti is a member of the Chancel Choir and the Soul Sisters. She also created the mission fund "Pass on Joy," which is designed to pass on joy to shut-ins and others who are in need of uplifting.

Together they manage the food truck "Twisted Flavors" owned by COHO LLC.

Misti and Jay are very proud of their three daughters, Lauren, Katie, and Anna. Lauren (Marc) Stringer has a degree in kinesiology from the University of Arkansas Fayetteville, a BSN from UAMS, and an MSN from UAMS. Katie (Tyler) Henderson has a psychology degree from the University of Arkansas and a Master's degree in counseling education from UALR. Anna has a crop science degree from the University of Arkansas and is currently receiving her Masters in soil fertility from LSU.

Jay and Misti love spending their extra time with their four-year-old grandson, Barrett.

Misti and Jay Coker with grandson Barrett

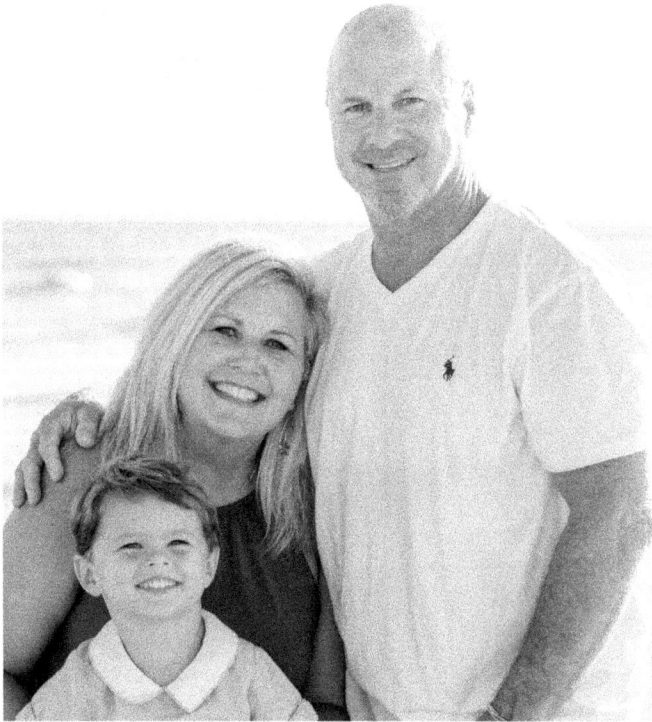

www.ingramcontent.com/pod-product-compliance
Lightning Source LLC
Chambersburg PA
CBHW071630200326

41519CB00012BA/2233